JUICING FOR BEGINNERS

A complete Guide to the Most Effective Juice Recipes for Weight
Loss, Body Cleansing, Energy Boosting and Skin Glow

SHERLIN FOSTER

TABLE OF CONTENTS

CHAPTER 5

CHAPTER 6

INTRODUCTION

Juices made with fruits and vegetables have a whole series of benefits. I have tried them for a long time and I have noticed their benefits; mainly I have lost weight and it has helped me with my stomach. With juices, you can achieve your health goals and you will increase your physical energy and your mental focus. I have tried that and I now want you to enjoy it. Another benefit they provide is that you can cleanse the body and detoxify yourself.

If you are not a person who has been consuming juices as a daily habit and trying different recipes for health, you are in the right place. Throughout the book, I will talk to you from the most basic concepts to preparing many recipes for various benefits. You will learn the advantages of each one and how to prepare them with suitable recipes for any fruit processor, from electric to manual, so they are easy to make and you can combine them. The other point that I will show you in the book is a table of fruits and vegetables with the nutrients of each one. If you are someone who likes to take control of the food you eat, consult the table and you will be able to make juices as you wish.

I will also talk to you about all the benefits of juicing fruits and vegetables and what you need to do to obtain them. In this book, you will be able to have support and guidance so that—combined with your purposes and juices—you can achieve the goals you have.

I will leave you with a series of recipe ideas with tips on how to save money so that you have fresh and quality fruit on hand. You will also learn how to take advantage of that leftover pulp at the end so that, instead of throwing it away, you can use it for many dishes—you can even make soup with it!

But that's not all, you can lose weight if you combine juicing with good lifestyle habits; you can start living a healthier lifestyle naturally with the consumption of fruits and vegetables. If you are just starting in the world of juices, you need a guide to start your healing process, and with the recipes in each of the sections of this book, you will be able to apply them to your diet.

You have the power to achieve your ideal size and remove any medical concerns. With this book, you will have a guide to support you on the path of healing. You will be able to do a juice cleanse, rejuvenate your skin and your life in general, and fight free radicals—and all while saving money, because I will leave you tips to achieve it.

If you are looking for an alternative to make the most of the vitamins and nutrients of your vegetables with all their guaranteed benefits, vegetable and fruit juices are an ideal option that allows you to eat your vegetables raw without altering them as a cooking characteristic. But what is the best combination to make a really tasty juice good for your body?

While vegetable juice is delicious on its own, it can also be too strong for some people, so it's always a good idea to add a bit of fruit to enhance its flavor. In its pages, I will show you some recipes that are delicious combined and you can enjoy them. Learn how to make them tastier by increasing their nutritional value. In this case, apples are an excellent pairing with green leafy vegetables; while oranges combine very well with those products that provide more beta-carotene, such as carrots. If you want to know how to make vegetable juice, this book is for you!

A juice extractor takes out the juice from fresh fruits or vegetables. This liquid contains most of the vitamins, minerals, and phytochemicals (phytonutrients) found in the fruit. However, whole fruits and vegetables also contain healthy fiber, which is lacking in most fruit juices.

According to the Mayo Clinic, some people believe that juices are better than consuming fruits and vegetables because the body has better absorption of nutrients and they free the digestive system from digesting fiber. They say that juicing can reduce the risk of cancer, boost the immune system, remove toxins from the body, aid digestion, and lose weight.

Find out on the following pages how to prepare delicious juices made mainly with vegetables and fruits but also combined with other healthy ingredients that will help in your process of recovering physical health.

CHAPTER 1

WHY YOU SHOULD MAKE JUICE

I want to share some of the benefits I found when I started to include juices in my life; I could see these changes in just a few days.

You Get More Nutrients and Energy During the Day

Many are looking for ways to increase their energy levels. Whether you're working long hours, caring for a family member, or going to school, everyone requires a little help getting through the day. That's where the juice comes in handy.

Juicing not only gives your body the nutrients it needs to work properly but also helps boost your energy levels, since the body doesn't have to work as hard to digest it.

If you are looking for a natural way to increase energy levels, drink natural juices. You'll be surprised at how much of a difference it can make.

It Supports the Immune System

The immune system is your body's natural defense against infection and disease. The more powerful it is, the more capable it is of repelling those unwanted intruders.

You can do several activities to boost your immune system, one of which is to eat fresh fruits and vegetables. Juicing is a great way to increase your intake of these nutrient-dense foods.

If you're looking for ways to boost your immune system, you can include some fresh juice each day. Your body will thank you!

It Alkalizes the Body

Drinking juices every day helps to neutralize the pH of your body. While you have the structure to maintain a slightly alkaline pH, today's diet and lifestyle choices often cause more acidity. Over time, this can lead to serious health problems.

When you add alkalizing fruits and vegetables to those juice drinks, you help offset the consumption of acidic foods and drinks. This helps protect your bones and teeth, improve digestion, reduce inflammation, and increase energy levels. So, if you want an easy way to improve your health, start adding more fresh juices to your diet!

It Delays Aging

Drinking freshly squeezed fruits and vegetables has great benefits for your health, including slowing down, and in some cases, even reversing the signs of aging. How does this work?

The body keeps in the fresh juice's nutrients as soon as you drink them so it can work with them, repairing damage and stimulating cell renewal. This helps to have healthy, rejuvenated, and radiant skin.

Fresh juices are rich in antioxidants, which help protect cells from harm caused by free radicals. Free radicals are to blame for premature aging, so, getting enough antioxidants can give you a youthful appearance. In addition, vitamins provide luminosity to the skin.

It Detoxifies the Organism

Eating freshly squeezed fruits and vegetables is one of the best actions you can do for your body. You are going to provide vitamins, minerals, and antioxidants; in addition, it helps to clean and purify your system.

One of the essential benefits of juices is that they serve to reduce toxins in the body. This is because the juice's nutrients serve to stimulate the liver and help with healthy digestion. In addition, juices can help purify toxins through the pores, improving the health of your skin.

It Helps You Lose Weight

Obesity is a huge problem that has led to an increase in chronic diseases such as type 2 diabetes, heart disease, and stroke. People are looking for new methods to lose weight, and one of the best ways to do it is to add natural ingredients to your diet.

One way to help with weight loss is juicing. It can help people lose weight by providing a calorie-controlled diet along with nutrients that promote satiety and help with weight loss. For example, one study found that participants who drank fresh-squeezed vegetable juice daily lost more weight than those who drank no juice at all.

It Provides Minerals and Vitamins to the Bloodstream

A healthy diet is key for many reasons, but did you know that what you eat also has an impact on your blood? That's right! The nutrients in food nourish the body, plus they are vital for maintaining blood flow. One way to make sure your blood gets the nutrients it needs is juicing.

Juice delivers minerals and vitamins that go directly into the blood, which helps it to flow well. Minerals like iron and copper are essential for building red blood cells, while vitamins like vitamin C keep blood vessels healthy. In addition, juices improve circulation by increasing the amount of oxygen in the blood.

It Helps Reduce High Levels of Bad Cholesterol and High Blood Pressure

The juice helps reduce bad cholesterol if it is at high levels and high blood pressure, two factors that can lead to serious health problems.

It's always a good idea to add fresh fruits and vegetables to your diet, but juicing helps make sure you're getting the nutrients that make up your diet. When you juice fruits and vegetables, vitamins, minerals, and antioxidants are more easily absorbed by the body. These nutrients help keep your heart healthy and prevent risks of cardiovascular problems. Not only do you find more of the healthy nutrients you need, but you also lower your cholesterol and blood pressure levels.

It Fights Eating Disorders

Eating disorders and other eating problems are related to physical and mental health issues. Overcoming diseases such as binge eating has become a serious problem. To stop overeating, you need regular eating habits. Therefore, including fruit juice in your diet can be a good deterrent to this condition. Including juices such as grapefruit can help overcome excess food.

It Helps Feel Physical and Mental Improvement

Daily juicing, including lots of fruits and vegetables, has many benefits. Juicing allows you to eat more fruits and vegetables each day than usual. This increased consumption has various health benefits, such as more favorable digestion, increased metabolism, and higher nutrient absorption.

In addition, the advantages found in the drinks allow you to delight in the delicious taste of fresh fruit juice. You can experiment with different mixes of flavors to find the ones you love. With so many tasty and nutritious options, there's no reason not to start juicing today! Let's not forget that in a few pages, you will have many recipes.

It Keeps Your Body Hydrated

Our bodies are mainly made up of water, so being hydrated is essential for your good health. When you drink juice, you are not just consuming fruits and vegetables, but the nutrients and vitamins required for proper hydration.

Juicing is a great way to boost your body to stay hydrated, especially if you're not good at drinking enough water throughout the day. Juices give your body the fluid it needs, but they will also eliminate toxins and contribute to healthy digestion.

Try to incorporate a little freshly squeezed juice into your daily life, as it is a good way to increase the body's hydration levels.

Juicing has wide-ranging benefits, including better digestion, more energy, detoxification, and clearer skin. Drinking juice is a great way to get nutrients to the body with something delicious and easy to consume. If you are looking for ways to improve your health, juicing is a great option.

Have you ever felt exhausted, bloated, or just couldn't control what you ate? Or perhaps you've struggled with health issues, whether mysterious or chronic, that just won't go away? I've been there, too!

Some time ago, I was diagnosed with carpal tunnel syndrome. I had so much pain in my wrist that it was very numb at night and I had trouble sleeping. I had to wear wrist splints, especially when lying down. After the second steroid injection was given to my wrist, I chose not to have a third injection.

I heard how fruit and vegetable juices could fill my body with nutrients and help improve my health, so I decided to give them a try.

Another time juicing came to my rescue was when I wanted to lose a few pounds. My ideal weight is 140 pounds, but sometimes the scale strays a bit from that number. So, I put myself on a juicing program to see what happens.

The results after drinking fruit and vegetable juices more frequently showed me that:

- I began to think more clearly.
- I lost a lot of weight, about a pound a day.
- I found myself with a lot of energy.
- I was more consistently positive, no matter what came my way.
- I woke up feeling fit and rested, even if I had slept less.
- The juices filled my system with so many nutrients that I rarely felt hungry.
- I also noticed an increase in smell and taste.
- My skin became brighter, and my hair and nails grew faster. People started commenting that I looked younger.
- My immune function was at its peak and I didn't catch a cold or get sick.
- The discipline of juicing gave me more control over my appetite and increased my overall will-power.

Given all these benefits, do you think it is worth drinking juices every day? You will see some recipes later, but for now, I want to leave you with some tips to keep in mind if you want to get serious about preparing juices.

CHAPTER 2
JUICING TIPS FOR BEGINNERS

As we saw in the previous chapter, there are several benefits of including natural juices every day, now I'll leave you some tips to keep in mind before starting to prepare them.

Recommended Juices per Day

Juice is healthy and tasty, but how much could you drink daily? The answer might seem unbelievable to you. Most health experts recommend drinking 64 ounces of water per day. However, when talking about natural juices, the recommendation is much lower. The juice boasts a variety of nutrients, including vitamins, minerals, and antioxidants, but since it's also high in sugar, it's best to limit your intake to no more than 16 ounces a day. Drinking too much juice could cause you to gain weight, as well as other health problems like diabetes and heart disease. If you want health improvements, make sure you drink juice in moderation.

Most of the juices have vegetable ingredients, with little fruit and herbs to give them a unique flavor. Some people believe that juice should not be sweet, but many people put fruit in it for flavor. The juice, as you saw before, has great health benefits, but its composition varies. The juice does not include all the nutrients and fiber we find in the raw ingredients. Even fruit juices that contain a lot of vegetables can give you a lot of sugar. Kidney stones can make emptying the intestines more difficult.

Types of Juicers on the Market and How to Choose the Best One

There are several types of juicers available in the market, each one with its own features and functionalities.

Let's see them and explain the qualities of each one of them:

Centrifugal Juicers:

These are the most common and affordable type of juicers. They work by chopping the fruit or vegetable with a flat cutting blade, then spinning the produce at a high speed to separate the juice from the pulp. They are an interesting option if you are starting in the world of juicers.

As a disadvantage, it could be said that they do not extract as much juice as other types of juicers and can make more noise, they are also a little more difficult to clean.

Masticating Juicers (Slow Juicers):

They are juicers that have a slow chewing movement so that you can extract the juice from vegetables and fruits. They are usually more expensive than centrifugal juicers, but you can get more juice and they have more nutrients.

This type of juicer makes less noise and is easier to clean than the previous ones; they can require more time and effort to use.

Citrus Juicers:

They are devices designed to extract juice from citrus fruits, such as limes, lemons, and oranges. They are usually the cheapest and using them is very simple. However, they are only limited to squeezing citrus and are not as versatile as other models.

Twin-Gear (Triturating) Juicers:

These are the most efficient and also the most expensive type of juicers. They have two gears that rotate inwards, grinding and crushing the fruit or vegetable to extract the juice. They are excellent at juicing a wide range of produce, including leafy greens, and they produce a very high-quality juice with minimal oxidation.

Press Juicers (Hydraulic Press Juicers):

These juicers extract juice by pressing fruit and vegetables under high pressure. They are known for their ability to produce a high yield of high-quality juice. However, they are often more expensive and require more effort to use than other types of juicers.

Industrial Juicers

They are the typical juicers we see in coffee shops. With the push of a button, we have quick and easy access to natural juice. Sadly, this will not count as a home juicer.

The best juicer for you depends on your specific needs, budget, and what you plan to juice. It's very important to consider these factors when choosing a juicer, that's why I prepare an easy quiz to help you making the right choice.

BONUS 1: Quiz to Help You Choose the Right Juicer for your Needs

When it comes to buy a juicer, you can really get confused from the number of models you will find in the stores.

Just by answering these few questions, your choice will not only be much easier and more informed, but it will also help you not to lose money or get wrong expectations from your juicer.

1. What is your budget for a new juicer?

A. Less than $100

B. $100 – $200

C. $200 – $400

D. $400 or more

2. **What do you plan to juice the most?**

A. Mostly citrus fruits

B. A variety of fruits and vegetables, including leafy greens

C. Mostly hard fruits and vegetables

D. A mix of everything, including citrus, hard produce, and leafy greens

3. **How important is the speed of juicing to you?**

A. Very important – I need my juice fast

B. Somewhat important – I don't want it to take forever

C. Not very important – I'm more concerned about juice quality

D. Not important at all – I'm willing to wait for the best juice

4. **How important is the noise level of the juicer?**

A. Very important – I need it to be quiet

B. Somewhat important – I don't want it to be too loud

C. Not very important – I don't mind a bit of noise

D. Not important at all – Noise doesn't bother me

5. **How important is the ease of cleaning to you?**

A. Very important – I want it to be easy to clean

B. Somewhat important – I don't want it to be too difficult to clean

C. Not very important – I don't mind spending some time cleaning

D. Not important at all – I'm willing to put in the effort to clean

6. **Are you interested in a juicer that can also make nut milk, sorbets, or other foods?**

A. Yes, definitely

B. Maybe, it could be a nice feature

C. Not really, I'm mostly interested in juicing

D. No, I only want to juice

7. **How important is the quality and nutritional value of the juice to you?**

   A. Very important – I want the highest quality juice

   B. Somewhat important – I want good quality juice, but it's not the only factor

   C. Not very important – I'm more concerned about other factors

   D. Not important at all – I just want juice, regardless of quality

8. **How much space do you have for a juicer?**

   A. Very little – I need a compact model

   B. Some – I can accommodate a medium-sized juicer

   C. A lot – I have plenty of counter space for any size juicer

   D. Space is not a concern for me

Here there are your answers:

1. **Mostly A's**: You are looking for a budget-friendly, fast, quiet, easy-to-clean juicer for mostly citrus fruits. They also value compactness. A **Citrus Juicer** would be a good fit for you. If you're planning to juice more than just citrus, a **Centrifugal Juicer** could also work, though it might be a bit louder.

2. **Mostly B's**: You are looking for a moderately priced juicer that can handle a variety of fruits and vegetables. You value a balance between speed and quality, don't mind some noise, and would like a juicer that's relatively easy to clean. You might also be interested in making nut milk or sorbets. A **Masticating Juicer** (also known as a slow juicer) would be a good fit for you.

3. **Mostly C's**: You are willing to invest more for a juicer that can handle mostly hard fruits and vegetables. You don't mind a slower juicing process or spending more time on cleaning. A **Centrifugal Juicer** could work for you, but you might also consider a **Masticating Juicer** for a higher juice yield and quality.

4. **Mostly D's**: You are willing to invest in a high-end juicer that can handle a mix of everything, including citrus, hard produce, and leafy greens. You don't mind a slower juicing process, some noise, or spending more time on cleaning. You're also interested in making other foods with their juicer, and you have plenty of space for a larger model. A **Twin-Gear (Triturating) Juicer** or a **Hydraulic Press Juicer** would be a good fit, offering the highest quality and versatility.

I hope that helped you, but remember, these are just general recommendations.

Importance of Organic Fruits and Vegetables

The benefits of organic fruit include a long list of properties for the health of consumers and producers, as well as for the protection of the environment. Organic fruit is a product elaborated through a process established by recognized standards, which includes avoiding the use of chemical fertilizers, pesticides, herbicides, hormones, genetically modified elements, and a host of other methods that can harm the environment.

Organic farming began long ago and has continued to evolve ever since, allowing new technologies to flourish and certifications to emerge in countries around the world.

What are the benefits of organic fruit? First, it protects the planet by reducing the number of harmful chemicals in the environment, which in turn, helps maintain soil fertility, cultivate in an environmentally friendly way, keep a conscious diet, and improve people's health, because, in many cases, pesticides have been linked to digestive problems, poisoning, and even anxiety.

It is also important to consider that organic fruits and vegetables contain high amounts of antioxidants and polyphenols, which work in the body to fight free radicals that directly affect cells.

Another great advantage is that this type of fruit contains more nutrients because it is a live product. It remains optimal for consumption for a longer time since the growth and development time of the plant is respected.

In addition to everything, since they are non-frozen products and without chemicals that change their state, they have a very special flavor.

What Fruits and Vegetables Should Not Be Juiced

All fruits and vegetables could be juiced, what should not be done is to combine some foods. For example, plums and pears provide too much fructose which ends up in something that would not be good for those who suffer from diabetes or are pre-diabetic.

These are some of the fruits that you shouldn't combine:

- Oranges and carrots: This combination increases stomach acid. So, if you suffer from this condition, I recommend not consuming it. Otherwise, you can drink it, but in moderation.
- Pineapple and dairy products: Pineapple contains an enzyme called bromelain, which can cause poisoning when mixed with milk, yogurt, etc. In general, acidic fruits should not be mixed with dairy products, as they can slow down digestion and make you feel heavy.
- Banana with milk: This mixture slows down digestion, which makes the body feel bad.
- Guava plus banana: This combination can create acidosis problems.
- Papaya with lemon: Although it is an unusual combination, the mixture of these fruits can cause blood complications, especially related to the amount of hemoglobin. Therefore, it can cause severe anemia.
- Plums and pears: This combination provides a high fructose content, so it is not recommended for diabetics.
- Oranges and lemons: If these two fruits are mixed in a big quantity, they can cause gastritis.
- Papaya and dragon fruit: Their combination can cause diarrhea.
- Avocado: Avocado is a fruit that has a lot of healthy fats, but it doesn't make good juice and can block the juicer.
- Coconut: Coconut is another fruit that doesn't juice well and can affect the motor of a juicer; use coconut water instead.
- Eggplant.
- Sweet potato.
- Seeds and pits: Such as cherry pits and apple seeds.

- Rhubarb: Rhubarb is a very fibrous and hard vegetable to juice effectively. It is also strong in oxalic acid, which can affect you in large amounts.
- Citrus zest (white part may be bitter) unless needed in a recipe.
- Kale stalks: While kale leaves are great for juicing, stalks don't juice as much and can also make the juice taste bitter.
- Broccoli.

It's important to remember that the fructose in fruit is the sugar your body needs to nourish your brain and pancreas, and when combined correctly, the fruit won't cause any kind of fermentation in your body. For this reason, it is imperative to create healthy combinations to help our bodies function better.

How to Store the Juices

If you want to keep fresh-squeezed juice longer without putting it in the freezer, you can keep it in the fridge for up to 3 days. If frozen, it will keep for 12–16 months.

What Is the Best Way to Preserve Natural Juices?

It will depend on how long you want to keep it and if you want to preserve its vitamins and nutrients. Storing juices in the fridge ensures that they contain fewer vitamins than they would at room temperature. Keeping natural juices in the freezer will help you store them longer and you'll lose fewer nutrients.

How Can I Get More Nutrients in My Fresh Juice?

When using fruit with edible skin, such as an apple, leave the skin on. The skin is rich in vitamins and nutrients, perfect for freshly squeezed juices. Adding the skin to the juice helps extend the shelf life of the vitamins and increases the nutritional profile of the drink.

In the next chapter, you will know the calories that some fruits and vegetables have per serving, so you can take them into account when you use some of them in juice recipes.

CHAPTER 3
BENEFITS OF FRUITS AND VEGETABLES AND TABLE OF NUTRIENTS

After learning how to preserve the juices and enjoy them, learn the table of nutrients for each of the ingredients.

Vegetables and fruits are foods that provide many benefits to our bodies since they contain vitamins and minerals necessary to maintain good health. Among its benefits, we can mention:

- Due to their fiber content, they favor adequate intestinal transit, as well as help to keep blood sugar levels more stable.
- They have an important antioxidant effect, mainly due to the vitamins and minerals they provide, which also allow us to have healthy skin.
- Phytochemicals found in vegetables and red fruits may improve heart health and reduce cancer risk.
- They help us lower cholesterol and blood pressure and prevent diabetes.

For the above reasons and many others, it is recommended to eat fruits and vegetables daily.

However, for obese patients, with triglyceride problems or people with diabetes, it is sometimes necessary to limit the intake of some fruits and vegetables.

Finally, it is worth mentioning that neither fruits nor vegetables are prohibited because they are natural, without added saturated fat, sodium, or sugar.

Here's a table listing the calorie and macronutrient (protein, carbohydrate, and fat lipid) contributions per 100 g of fruits and vegetables, all of which are classified as allowable intakes, but their carbohydrates are ranked by intake from low to high.

Nutritional Table of Fruits

FOOD (100 G)	CALORIES	PROTEINS	CARBS	FATS
Acai	70 kcal	0.8 g	6 g	12 g
Apple	52 kcal	0.3 g	14 g	0.3 g
Apricot	48 kcal	0.5 g	3.9 g	0.1 g

FOOD (100 G)	CALORIES	PROTEINS	CARBS	FATS
Avocado	160 kcal	2 g	1.9 g	15 g
Banana	89 kcal	1.1 g	23 g	0.3 g
Blackberries	43 kcal	1.4 g	9.6 g	0.5 g
Blueberries	57 kcal	0.7 g	14 g	0.3 g
Cantaloupe melon	34 kcal	0.8 g	8.2 g	0.2 g
Cherries	50 kcal	1.1 g	12 g	0.2 g
Clementine	47 kcal	1 g	12 g	0.2 g
Compote/ Apple puree	68 kcal	0.3 g	10 g	0.1 g
Dates	282 kcal	2 g	75 g	0.2 g
Figs	74 kcal	0.9 g	19 g	0.3 g
Gallic melon	26 kcal	0.8 g	8 g	0.2 g
Gooseberry	56 kcal	1 g	8 g	0.2 g
Grapefruit	42 kcal	0.8 g	8 g	0.1 g
Grapes	69 kcal	0.6 g	18 g	0.2 g
Green plum	41 kcal	0.5 g	9.5 g	0.3 g
Grenade	83 kcal	1.7 g	18.7 g	1.2 g
Guava	68 kcal	2.6 g	14.3 g	1 g
Jackfruit	95 kcal	1.5 g	24 g	0.3 g
Kiwi	61 kcal	1.1 g	14.7 g	0.5 g
Lemon	29 kcal	1.1 g	9.3 g	0.3 g
Lime	30 kcal	0.7 g	10.5 g	0.2 g
Lychee	66 kcal	0.8 g	17 g	0.4 g

FOOD (100 G)	CALORIES	PROTEINS	CARBS	FATS
Macedonian	50 kcal	0.9 g	11 g	0.3 g
Mango	60 kcal	0.8 g	14.9 g	0.4 g
Melon	36 kcal	0.8 g	8.1 g	0.2 g
Nectarine	44 kcal	0.9 g	10.6 g	0.3 g
Olives	115 kcal	0.8 g	3.8 g	15.3 g
Orange	47 kcal	1.2 g	11.8 g	0.2 g
Papaya	43 kcal	0.5 g	10.8 g	0.3 g
Passion fruit	97 kcal	2.2 g	23.4 g	0.7 g
Peach	39 kcal	0.9 g	9.5 g	0.3 g
Pear	57 kcal	0.4 g	15.5 g	0.3 g
Persimmon	127 kcal	0.6 g	18.6 g	0.4 g
Physalis	49 kcal	1 g	11.2 g	1 g
Pineapple	50 kcal	0.5 g	13.1 g	0.1 g
Plantain	122 kcal	1.3 g	22.8 g	0.3 g
Plum	46 kcal	0.6 g	11.4 g	0.3 g
Prickly pear	37 kcal	0.7 g	9.6 g	0.5 g
Quince	57 kcal	0.4 g	15.3 g	0.1 g
Raisins	299 kcal	3.1 g	79.2 g	0.5 g
Rambutan	82 kcal	0.9 g	20.9 g	0.2 g
Raspberry	52 kcal	1.2 g	11.9 g	0.7 g
Red orange	50 kcal	1 g	8.2 g	0.2 g
Rhubarb	21 kcal	0.9 g	3.2 g	0.2 g
Star fruit	31 kcal	1 g	6.7 g	0.3 g

FOOD (100 G)	CALORIES	PROTEINS	CARBS	FATS
Strawberries	32 kcal	0.8 g	7.7 g	0.3 g
Tamarind	239 kcal	2.8 g	62.5 g	0.6 g
Tangerine	53 kcal	0.8 g	13.3 g	0.3 g
Watermelon	30 kcal	0.6 g	7.6 g	0.2 g
Yellow melon	55 kcal	0.8 g	8.2 g	0.2 g

Nutritional Table of Vegetables

FOOD (100 G)	CALORIES	PROTEINS	CARBS	FATS
Artichoke	47 kcal	3.3 g	11.4 g	0.2 g
Asparagus	20 kcal	2.2 g	3.7 g	0.2 g
Beet	43 kcal	1.6 g	9.6 g	0.2 g
Bell pepper	23 kcal	1 g	4.6 g	0.3 g
Broccoli	34 kcal	2.8 g	6.6 g	0.4 g
Brussels sprouts	43 kcal	3.4 g	8.9 g	0.3 g
Cabbage	25 kcal	1.3 g	5.8 g	0.2 g
Carrot	41 kcal	0.9 g	10 g	0.2 g
Cauliflower	25 kcal	1.9 g	5 g	0.3 g
Celery	16 kcal	0.7 g	2.9 g	0.2 g
Chard	19 kcal	1.8 g	3.7 g	0.2 g
Cherry tomato	100 kcal	1 g	3.9 g	0.2 g
Chicory	72 kcal	1.7 g	4.7 g	0.3 g
Chinese cabbage	16 kcal	1.2 g	2.2 g	0.2 g
Chives	30 kcal	2 g	4.4 g	0.5 g

FOOD (100 G)	CALORIES	PROTEINS	CARBS	FATS
Collards/ Green cabbage	32 kcal	3.3 g	5.6 g	0.7 g
Corn	98 kcal	3.2 g	18.7 g	1.2 g
Corn grains	365 kcal	3.3 g	24.5 g	1.4 g
Cucumber	16 kcal	0.6 g	3.6 g	0.1 g
Eggplant	25 kcal	1 g	5.7 g	0.2 g
Endive	17 kcal	1.3 g	3.4 g	0.2 g
Fennel/Dill	31 kcal	1.2 g	7.3 g	0.2 g
Garlic	149 kcal	6.4 g	29.9 g	0.5 g
Green beans	31 kcal	1.8 g	7.9 g	0.2 g
Green bell pepper	28 kcal	1 g	4.6 g	0.3 g
Green onion	32 kcal	1.8 g	7.3 g	0.2 g
Green tomato	23 kcal	1.2 g	5.1 g	0.2 g
Horseradish	48 kcal	1.2 g	11.3 g	0.7 g
Italian Pepper/ Frying Pepper	23 kcal	1.2 g	2.6 g	0.3 g
Kale	49 kcal	4.3 g	8.8 g	0.7 g
Leek	61 kcal	1.5 g	14.2 g	0.3 g
Lettuce	15 kcal	1.4 g	2.9 g	0.2 g
Lupins	120 kcal	36.3 g	40.1 g	9.7 g
Mushrooms/ Fungi	22 kcal	3.1 g	3.3 g	0.3 g
Mustard grains/ leaves	27 kcal	2.7 g	6 g	0.4 g

FOOD (100 G)	CALORIES	PROTEINS	CARBS	FATS
Nori/Seaweed nori	35 kcal	5.8 g	5.1 g	0.2 g
Okra	33 kcal	2 g	7.5 g	0.2 g
Olives/Black olives/ Green olives	115 kcal	0.8 g	6 g	10.7 g
Onion	40 kcal	1.1 g	9.3 g	0.1 g
Parsnips/ White turnips	75 kcal	1.2 g	17.6 g	0.3 g
Peas/ Chickpeas	81 kcal	9 g	60 g	6 g
Pepper	18 kcal	1 g	4.6 g	0.3 g
Pepper/Chili	27 kcal	1.9 g	9.5 g	0.4 g
Pickle	14 kcal	0.6 g	3.2 g	0.1 g
Piquillo pepper	22 kcal	1 g	5.3 g	0.3 g
Potato	77 kcal	2 g	17.6 g	0.1 g
Prickly pear	16 kcal	0.7 g	9.6 g	0.5 g
Pumpkin	14 kcal	1 g	6.5 g	0.1 g
Pumpkin	26 kcal	1 g	6.5 g	0.1 g
Radishes	16 kcal	0.7 g	3.4 g	0.1 g
Red bell pepper	35 kcal	1 g	4.6 g	0.3 g
Red cabbage	31 kcal	1.4 g	7.4 g	0.2 g
Red onion	40 kcal	1.1 g	9.3 g	0.1 g
Rocket/ Arugula	25 kcal	2.6 g	3.7 g	0.7 g

FOOD (100 G)	CALORIES	PROTEINS	CARBS	FATS
Shallots/ Purple onion	72 kcal	2.5 g	16.8 g	0.1 g
Spinach	23 kcal	2.9 g	3.6 g	0.4 g
Spinach cream	74 kcal	2.2 g	4.4 g	0.2 g
Squash	22 kcal	1.2 g	3.1 g	0.2 g
Swede	27 kcal	0.9 g	8.6 g	0.2 g
Swedish turnip	38 kcal	0.9 g	8.6 g	0.2 g
Sweet potato	86 kcal	1.6 g	20.1 g	0.1 g
Tomato	18 kcal	0.9 g	3.9 g	0.2 g
Turnip greens	20 kcal	1.5 g	4.4 g	0.3 g
Turnips	28 kcal	0.9 g	6.2 g	0.2 g
Wasabi	109 kcal	4.8 g	23.5 g	0.6 g
Yellow bell pep-per	19 kcal	1 g	6 g	0.2 g
Zucchini/ Courgettes	17 kcal	1.2 g	3.1 g	0.2 g

Now that you have seen each food has different calories, in the next chapter, we will start with the first recipes for you to flatten your belly and lose weight.

CHAPTER 4

BELLY FLATTENING JUICE RECIPES

Raspberry, Apple, and Orange

INGREDIENTS FOR 2-3 GLASSES OF JUICE

- 1 green apple
- Water (a little)
- 20 raspberries
- 3 oranges

PREPARATION

1. Peel and slice the apples.
2. Add the apples, raspberries, and water to the blender jar and blend.
3. Squeeze the orange, strain the juice, add it to the glass, and continue stirring.
4. Pour some more water if you think it's necessary.
5. Strain the juice to remove the raspberry seeds, and voila!

Calories: Approximately 190-220 calories
Carbohydrates: Around 45-55 grams
Protein: Roughly 3-4 grams
Fat: Negligible amount
Fiber: About 12-15 grams
Vitamin C: Significant amount from the oranges
Antioxidants: High content from raspberries and oranges

It is ideal to drink this antioxidant juice every morning on an empty stomach for a full week to lose weight fast. Thanks to the ketones that make up raspberry, it is possible to lose weight quickly and see results in a short time.

Melon and Mint Juice to Reduce Inflammation

INGREDIENTS FOR 2-3 GLASSES OF JUICE

- ½ small Chinese melon
- 1 lemon, peeled
- 1 small cucumber
- 1 cup seedless green grapes
- A small bunch of mint

PREPARATION

1. Wash and clean all components.
2. Pour them into the extractor. If you're using a blender, add a cup of water to help mix the ingredients.

Calories: Approximately 130-160 calories
Carbohydrates: Around 30-40 grams
Protein: Roughly 2-3 grams

Fat: Negligible amount
Fiber: About 4-6 grams
Vitamin C: Significant amount from the lemon
Potassium: Present from the melon, cucumber, and grapes
Antioxidants: Present in the melon, grapes, lemon, and mint

All the ingredients in this recipe have great diuretic and digestive properties, they are good for reducing inflammation in the body and creating a feeling of lightness.

Cleansing Juice

INGREDIENTS FOR APPROXIMATELY 1-2 GLASSES OF JUICE

- 10 mint leaves
- 100 g (3.5 oz) raspberries
- 100 g (3.5 oz) strawberries
- 5 basil leaves
- 50 g (1.7 oz) blueberries

PREPARATION

1. To prepare it, start the juicer by hand and place the washed fruit and green leaves inside it.
2. If you want this preparation to have an additional, you can take frozen berries and if the juicer has it, put the filter on it, so your juice will become a refreshing and purifying frozen sorbet.
3. Ideal for hot days, although if not, simply squeeze and pass through a strainer.

Calories: 80-100 calories
Carbohydrates: 18-22 grams
Protein: 1-2 grams
Fat: 0-1 gram

Fiber: 5-6 grams
Vitamin C: Provides a significant amount from the raspberries and strawberries

Antioxidants: Found in the berries and basil leaves

Juice to Clean

INGREDIENTS FOR 1-2 GLASSES OF JUICE

- ½ cucumber
- ½ cup pineapple chunks
- 1 green apple
- 1 cup spinach
- 2 celery stalks

PREPARATION

1. For you to have juice that cleanses and flattens the belly like this, you only have to cut the fruits and vegetables to the appropriate size for your juice.
2. You will not have to worry about the pulp since you can choose how much of it you want to put.
3. Some models of juicers have a filter to obtain a juice with a smooth or thicker texture, it depends on what you like.
4. After you collect the juice in the jug of your extractor, you can give it more strength with a superfood like spirulina powder, which is rich in essential fatty acids, vitamins, and minerals.

Calories: 120-150 calories
Carbohydrates: 25-30 grams
Protein: 2-3 grams
Fat: 1 gram

Fiber: 6-8 grams
Vitamin C: Significant amount from the pineapple and apple
Vitamin A: Provided by

the spinach and celery
Potassium: Present from the cucumber, pineapple, apple, and celery

Pineapple and Ginger

INGREDIENTS FOR APPROXIMATELY 2-3 GLASSES OF JUICE

- 1 orange
- 2 cups pineapple chunks
- A small piece of ginger

PREPARATION

1. Start the juicer to process the pineapple, so you will get all the juice out of it.
2. Do the same with the orange and combine. When finished, add a little grated ginger and enjoy.

Calories: 180-220 calories
Carbohydrates: 45-55 grams
Protein: 2-3 grams
Fat: 1 gram

Fiber: 4-6 grams
Vitamin C: Significant amount from the orange and pineapple
Vitamin A: Provided by the

orange and pineapple
Potassium: Present from the pineapple and orange

Gingerol: Antioxidant and anti-inflammatory properties from the ginger

Orange Juice With a Spicy Touch

INGREDIENTS FOR 2-3 GLASSES OF JUICE

- ½ small pineapple
- 1 piece of ginger (1 cm), peeled
- 1 peeled carrot
- 2 peeled clementines

PREPARATION

1. Cut the carrot and pineapple into pieces according to the size of your juicer and put them inside.
2. Add the clementines and ginger.
3. Squeeze everything out and then place it in a large glass and serve.

Calories: 140-170 calories
Carbohydrates: 35-45 grams
Protein: 2-3 grams
Fat: 0 grams

Fiber: 4-6 grams
Vitamin C: Significant amount from the clementines and pineapple

Vitamin A: Provided by the carrot and pineapple
Potassium: Present from the pineapple and clementines

Gingerol: Antioxidant and anti-inflammatory properties from the ginger

Cucumber, Apple, and Spinach Juice

Start your day burning fat with an all-natural juice packed with cucumber, apple, and spinach. Get all the nutritional values, drink its pulp and all.

INGREDIENTS FOR APPROXIMATELY 1-2 GLASSES OF JUICE

- 1 large celery, chopped
- 1 handful of spinach
- 150 ml unsweetened apple juice, cold
- 5 cm (1.9 in) chopped cucumber
- Iced coconut water, optional
- Lime juice

PREPARATION

1. Put the vegetables in the juicer and process them.
2. Then, in a deep container, put the apple and lime juice and combine everything by hand until it is as smooth as possible.
3. Pour into a glass and drink as is or you can dilute with water to get the consistency you want.

Calories: 80-100 calories
Carbohydrates: 18-22 grams
Protein: 1-2 grams
Fat: 0 grams

Fiber: 3-4 grams
Vitamin A: Provided by the spinach and apple
Vitamin C: Present in the

apple and lime juice
Potassium: Provided by the celery, cucumber, and apple

Tip: After making this recipe, your extractor or juicer may be quite dirty compared to another preparation; clean thoroughly.

Fennel, Cranberry, and Apple Juice

Fruit and vegetable juices jump-start your body early. They're packed with nutrients like folic acid, fiber, and vitamin C.

INGREDIENTS FOR 1-2 GLASSES OF JUICE

- 1 small fennel bulb
- 1 tsp lemon juice
- 1 apple
- 85 g blueberries

PREPARATION

1. Trim the top and bottom of the fennel bulb and chop it into pieces.
2. Put the frozen fennel, apple, and cranberries in the juicer.
3. Process it as you would any food, then add lemon juice and serve immediately.

Calories: 80-100 calories
Carbohydrates: 18-22 grams
Protein: 1-2 grams

Fat: 0 grams
Fiber: 3-4 grams
Vitamin C: Provided by the

apple and lemon juice
Folic Acid: Present in the fennel and blueberries

Spinach and Broccoli Juice

Combine healthy ingredients like these for an energizing breakfast. Using unsweetened brown rice milk fortified with calcium and vitamins makes it more delicious and healthier.

INGREDIENTS FOR 1-2 GLASSES OF JUICE

- ¼ tsp spirulina or 1 tbsp vegetable powder or vegan protein powder (optional)
- 1 banana
- 1 handful of spinach (about 50 g/2 oz)
- 100 g broccoli chopped into small pieces
- 2 celery sticks
- 300 ml rice milk (or common milk)
- 4 tbsp desiccated coconut

PREPARATION

1. Place the spinach, celery, banana, and broccoli in the juicer and process.
2. Then add 300 ml water, the rice milk, and the tablespoons of coconut and mix until smooth.
3. Put the spirulina and the vegetable powder, mix again, and enjoy.

Calories: 200-250 calories
Carbohydrates: 35-40 grams
Protein: 8-10 grams (may vary depending on optional protein powder)

Fat: 6-8 grams
Fiber: 8-10 grams
Folic Acid: Provided by rice milk
Vitamin C: Provided by spinach and broccoli

Vitamin A: Provided by spinach and broccoli

Low-Sugar Lime and Basil Green Juice

This is an aromatic and flavorful lime and basil juice very easy to prepare. You can make this refreshing drink in minutes. The greens and a dash of elderflower sweetness give it a unique twist.

INGREDIENTS FOR APPROXIMATELY 1 GLASS OF JUICE

- 1 lime, grated and squeezed
- 20 g (0.7 oz) basil leaves
- 50 g (1.7 oz) baby spinach
- 70 ml apple juice
- A 6-cm (2.3 in) cucumber piece (about 100 g/3.5 oz), chopped

PREPARATION

1. Squeeze the cucumber and place it in a jar. Add the apple juice to a large pitcher, then the spinach, basil, lime, and 100 ml cold water.
2. Put it in a glass and drink immediately.

Calories: Approximately 70-90 calories
Carbohydrates: Around 15-20 grams
Protein: Approximately 1-2 grams

Fat: Negligible amount
Fiber: About 3-5 grams
Vitamin C: Provided by lime and spinach
Vitamin A: Provided by spinach

Folic Acid: Present in spinach and basil
Iron: Present in spinach and basil

Sweet Melon, Cucumber, and Lime Juice

This sparkling green-hued drink comes packed with a wealth of fresh ingredients to leave you feeling refreshed and energized.

INGREDIENTS FOR APPROXIMATELY 1 GLASS OF JUICE

- ¼ large sweet melon
- ½ cucumber, cut into large pieces
- 1 lime

PREPARATION

1. Take the melon, scoop out the seeds, and then mince the pulp from the outer skin and chop it into chunks.
2. Put the melon, cucumber, and lime in the juicer and process it.
3. Pour into a glass and serve.

Calories: Approximately 60-80 calories
Carbohydrates: Around 15-20 grams
Protein: Approximately 1 gram

Fat: Negligible amount
Fiber: About 2-4 grams
Vitamin C: Provided by lime and sweet melon
Potassium: Present in sweet

melon and cucumber
Vitamin A: Present in sweet melon
Vitamin K: Present in cucumber

Delicious Juice to Start the Body and Burn Fat

Berries can go hand in hand with energy and fat burning, you will see how delicious this recipe is.

INGREDIENTS FOR 1 GLASS OF JUICE

- 1 small ripe banana
- Apple juice or mineral water
- Honey (optional)
- 140 g (4.9 oz) blackberries, blueberries, raspberries, or strawberries

PREPARATION

1. Cut the banana, put it in the juicer, and add the berries of your choice.
2. Beat until smooth. You can add juice or water to get the consistency you want.
3. Put some additional fruits on top. Add honey and serve.

Calories: Approximately 150-200 calories
Carbohydrates: Around 35-45 grams

Protein: Approximately 2-3 grams
Fat: Negligible amount
Fiber: About 6-8 grams
Vitamin C: Provided by the berries

Potassium: Present in the banana and berries
Antioxidants: Present in the berries

Strawberry, Banana, and Orange Juice

Have a good dose of fruit with this banana and orange recipe. It's dairy-free so you won't have those extra calories for your weight, making it a great start to anyone's day.

INGREDIENTS FOR APPROXIMATELY 1 GLASS OF JUICE

- 1 small banana, sliced
- 10 strawberries, peeled (approximately 175 g/6.17 oz)
- 100 ml orange juice

PREPARATION

1. Combine the strawberries with the banana in the juicer.
2. Then, add the orange juice and process it until smooth.
3. Pour the smoothie into a glass and enjoy.

Calories: Approximately 120-150 calories
Carbohydrates: Around 28-35 grams
Protein: Approximately 1-2 grams

Fat: Negligible amount
Fiber: About 4-6 grams
Vitamin C: Provided by the strawberries and orange juice
Potassium: Present in the banana and strawberries

Antioxidants: Provided by the strawberries and orange juice

Açaí Smoothie

Açaí is a very good ingredient, with a reputation for being one of the best antioxidants, it is perfect for you to prepare it with pineapple, strawberries, and banana.

INGREDIENTS FOR APPROXIMATELY 2 TALL GLASSES OF THE AÇAÍ SMOOTHIE

- 1 medium banana
- 1 tbsp honey
- 100 g (3.5 oz) raw açaí pulp
- 100 g (3.5 oz) strawberry
- 250 ml mango or orange juice
- 50 g (0.7 oz) frozen pineapple

PREPARATION

1. Put all the ingredients in the juicer.
2. Process until smooth. If you see it very thick, add a little more mango or orange juice.

Calories: Approximately 250-300 calories per serving
Carbohydrates: Around 60-70 grams per serving
Protein: Approximately

2-4 grams per serving
Fat: Negligible amount Fiber: About 6-8 grams per serving
Vitamin C: Provided by the strawberries and citrus juice

Potassium: Present in the banana and açaí pulp
Antioxidants: Provided by the açaí pulp and strawberries

Sun Shake

You can start the day with a little ray of sunshine: this low–fat juice is loved by those who want to lose weight!

INGREDIENTS FOR APPROXIMATELY 2 GLASSES OF SHAKE

- 2 bananas
- 20 g (0.7 oz) nuts
- 200 g (7 oz) pineapple
- Lime juice
- 500 ml carrot juice
- A few pieces of ginger

PREPARATION

1. Place all the solid ingredients except the ginger in the juicer and process them.
2. Now add the liquid ingredients and grate some ginger on top before drinking.

Calories: Approximately 300-350 calories per serving
Carbohydrates: Around 60-70 grams per serving
Protein: Approximately 5-7 grams per serving

Fat: Around 10-12 grams per serving (mostly from the nuts)
Fiber: About 8-10 grams per serving
Vitamin C: Provided by the pineapple and lime juice

Vitamin A: Present in the carrot juice
Potassium: Provided by the bananas and pineapple
Healthy Fats: Provided by the nuts

Smoothies With Kale

Get a dose of vitamin C right off the bat with this vegan juice. Here we mix the kale with a little pineapple and spicy lemon.

INGREDIENTS FOR APPROXIMATELY 1-2 GLASSES OF SMOOTHIE

- ½ lime
- 1 tbsp nuts
- 1 pineapple
- 1 banana (optional)
- 2 handfuls of kale
- Ginger in medium size pieces

PREPARATION

1. Place all the ingredients except the ginger in the juicer and process them.
2. When finished, serve in a glass and enjoy after adding a little grated ginger.

Calories: Approximately 200-250 calories per serving
Carbohydrates: Around 40-50 grams per serving
Protein: Approximately 3-5 grams per serving (mostly from the nuts)

Fat: Around 2-4 grams per serving (mostly from the nuts)
Fiber: About 8-10 grams per serving
Vitamin C: Provided by the lime and pineapple

Vitamin A: Present in the kale
Potassium: Provided by the pineapple and banana (if used)
Healthy Fats: Provided by the nuts

Persimmon and Apple Juice

INGREDIENTS FOR 1-2 GLASSES OF JUICE

- 2 persimmons
- 2 apples
- A little bit of water

PREPARATION

1. The persimmon is a sweet autumn fruit. In some places, it is known as Palo de Santo. It has beta-carotene, provitamin A, vitamin C, B1, B2 and minerals (its potassium content stands out), and flavonoids (lycopene).
2. You can try consuming the persimmon in juice and you will see that you will like it.
3. You only need to put the persimmons and apples in the juicer, process, and serve, you can add water to taste until it has the desired consistency.

Calories: Approximately 150-200 calories per serving
Carbohydrates: Around 35-45 grams per serving
Protein: Approximately

1-2 grams per serving
Fat: Negligible amount
Fiber: About 5-7 grams per serving
Vitamin A: Provided by the

persimmons (beta-carotene)
Vitamin C: Provided by the persimmons and apples
Potassium: Present in the persimmons and apples

Juice to Lose Fat

Drinking fruit juice is a very healthy habit for the body. This kind of juice must be taken on an empty stomach to help eliminate fat. By containing antioxidants and vitamin C, they will be our allies to improve the immune system. It has a great taste, and no added sugar is required.

INGREDIENTS FOR 1-2 GLASSES OF JUICE

- 1 lemon
- 1 cucumber
- 2 juice oranges
- Parsley

PREPARATION

1. Place the cucumber in the processor and process, then place the oranges if you have not squeezed them, and the lemon—all separated.
2. When you have each liquid food, combine them. You can put a little parsley to garnish and give it an additional delicious flavor.

Calories: Approximately 70-100 calories per serving
Carbohydrates: Around 18-25 grams per serving
Protein: Approximately 2-3 grams per serving
Fat: Negligible amount
Fiber: About 4-6 grams per serving
Vitamin C: Provided by the lemon and oranges
Potassium: Present in the cucumber and oranges
Antioxidants: Provided by the lemon, cucumber, and oranges

Green Juice

Green juice is one of the most famous recipes for extractors. This recipe combines several fruits and vegetables for an explosion of flavor and a large amount of nutrients.

INGREDIENTS FOR 1-2 GLASSES OF JUICE

- 2 carrots
- 1 lemon
- ½ cucumber
- ½ apple
- ¼ fresh ginger

PREPARATION

1. Place the peeled carrots in the juicer and process.
2. Repeat the same with the lemon, apple, and cucumber and process them until you have juices that you will later combine.
3. Add the fresh ginger and serve.

Calories: Approximately 100-120 calories per serving
Carbohydrates: Around 25-30 grams per serving
Protein: Approximately 1-2 grams per serving
Fat: Negligible amount
Fiber: About 5-7 grams per serving
Vitamin C: Provided by the lemon
Vitamin A: Provided by the carrots
Potassium: Present in the cucumber

"Kill Kilograms" Vegetable Juice

This rich juice is highly diuretic and helps eliminate the residual liquid that we later confuse with "fatty" or "heavier" that we "feel" due to the high amounts of processed salt, glutamate, etc. we find in processed foods.

Plus, it's super detoxifying, with tons of vitamin C from lemon and pineapple, which boosts our defenses! Also, cucumbers keep us hydrated and spinach alkalizes and energizes us—it has everything, without a doubt.

This is the wonder of vegetables... one consumes them for a purpose and it turns out that it benefits us in 1000 other things. Nature is admirable, intelligent, and nutritious... we can also digest and process it... that's why it's natural.

INGREDIENTS FOR 1 OR 2 GLASSES OF JUICE

- 1 cup pineapple, without skin and chopped in pieces that fit in the juicer
- A celery stalk with everything and leaves
- 1 peeled cucumber
- 1 spinach
- 1 lemon, without the peel, just the white layer

PREPARATION

1. Take each of the ingredients to the juicer and process until its juice is obtained. Serve in a glass as it is; don't add sweeteners.
2. It can be taken 3 times a week, the rest you can combine with other juices.

Calories: Approximately 80-100 calories per serving
Carbohydrates: Around 20-25 grams per serving
Protein: Approximately 2-3 grams per serving
Fat: Negligible amount
Fiber: About 4-6 grams per serving
Vitamin C: Provided by the pineapple and lemon
Potassium: Present in the pineapple, celery, and cucumber

Pineapple and Mint Juice

In this recipe, you will find a refreshing combination of pineapple and mint with a hint of ginger. Perfect for those looking for a refreshing drink and an energy boost.

INGREDIENTS FOR 1-2 GLASSES OF JUICE

- 1 bunch of mint
- ½ lemon
- ½ pineapple
- A ½-cm fresh ginger piece

PREPARATION

1. Place the lemon and pineapple in the juicer and process them; then add the squeezed mint as well.
2. Serve with some fresh ginger on top.

Calories: Approximately 80-100 calories per serving
Carbohydrates: Around 20-25 grams per serving
Protein: Approximately 1-2 grams per serving
Fat: Negligible amount
Fiber: About 3-5 grams per serving
Vitamin C: Provided by the lemon and pineapple
Potassium: Present in the pineapple

Cranberry and Apple Juice

It is a recipe where sweet and sour flavors are combined. The cranberry apple juice is perfect for those who want a refreshing and healthy drink.

- 1 apple
- ½ lemon
- ½ cup water
- ½ cup blueberries

PREPARATION

1. Place the blueberries, apple, and lemon in the juicer and process.
2. Add ½ cup of water, mix and serve.

Calories: Approximately 80-100 calories per serving
Carbohydrates: Around 20-25 grams per serving

Protein: Approximately 1 gram per serving
Fat: Negligible amount
Fiber: About 3-5 grams

per serving
Vitamin C: Provided by the lemon
Antioxidants: Present in the blueberries and cranberries

Beetroot and Orange Juice

This juice refreshingly combines beetroot and orange. The beet can give you a large amount of nutrients, while the orange offers you a touch of sweet flavor.

INGREDIENTS FOR 1-2 GLASSES OF JUICE

- 1 lemon
- 1 beetroot
- ¼ fresh ginger
- 3 oranges

PREPARATION

1. Place the beets and oranges in the juicer and process.
2. Add the squeezed lemon and serve with a little ginger on top.

Calories: Approximately 150-200 calories per serving
Carbohydrates: Around 30-40 grams per serving

Protein: Approximately 3-5 grams per serving
Fat: Negligible amount
Fiber: About 5-8 grams

per serving
Vitamin C: Provided by the oranges and lemon
Folate:: Provided by the beetroot

CHAPTER 5
DETOX AND BODY CLEANSING JUICE RECIPES

After seeing the recipes to lower the belly, these are some for you to cleanse your body.

Kale and Pineapple Detox Smoothie

INGREDIENTS

- ½ can (16 oz) coconut milk
- ½ cup chopped kale
- 1 ½ cups fresh pineapple chunks
- 1 banana

PREPARATION

1. Put pineapple, banana, and kale in a juicer and process.
2. Serve with coconut milk.
3. Serving Size: 1 glass (approx. 8–10 oz)

Calories: 230-250
Total Fat: 13-15g
Saturated Fat: 11-12g

Cholesterol: 0mg
Sodium: 23-25mg
Total Carbohydrate: 29-31g

Dietary Fiber: 4-5g
Sugars: 17-19g
Protein: 2-3g

Mint, Spinach, and Bananas Green Smoothie

INGREDIENTS

- ½ cup packed fresh spinach
- ½ cup frozen sliced banana
- ½ cup green tea, cold
- 1 tbsp vanilla protein powder
- 1 tbsp chopped fresh mint
- 8 fl oz coconut water

PREPARATION

1. Combine banana, spinach, and mint and process them one by one in the juicer.
2. Add the coconut water and tea, along with the protein. Serve it.
3. Serving Size: 1 glass (approx. 8–10 oz)

Calories: 150-170
Total Fat: 1-2g
Saturated Fat: 0-1g

Cholesterol: 0mg
Sodium: 100-150mg
Total Carbohydrate: 33-35g

Dietary Fiber: 4-5g
Sugars: 19-21g
Protein: 4-5g

Green Goddess Juice

INGREDIENTS

- 3 celery stalks
- 1 medium green apple, cut into eighths
- 1 medium pear, cut into eighths
- ½ large cucumber, cut into quarters

PREPARATION

1. Squeeze all the ingredients one by one and then place them in a glass.
2. Drink immediately, or let it chill for an hour and then enjoy.
3. Serving Size: 1 glass (approx. 8–10 oz)

Calories: 70-90
Total Fat: 0-0.5g
Saturated Fat: 0g

Cholesterol: 0mg
Sodium: 40-60mg
Total Carbohydrate: 18-20g

Dietary Fiber: 3-4g
Sugars: 13-15g
Protein: 1g

Ginger Zinger Juice

INGREDIENTS

- A ½-inch fresh ginger piece
- ¼ lemon, peel removed to avoid bitterness
- 2 medium apples, cut into eighths
- 5 carrots (no need to peel them)

PREPARATION

1. Squeeze each of the ingredients in your juicer, place this mix in a glass, and put it in the refrigerator.
2. If you want to drink it fresh, consume it immediately.
3. Serving Size: 1 glass (approx. 8–10 oz)

Calories: 150-180
Total Fat: 0-0.5g
Saturated Fat: 0g

Cholesterol: 0mg
Sodium: 100-120mg
Total Carbohydrate: 38-42g

Dietary Fiber: 6-8g
Sugars: 28-32g
Protein: 1-2g

Tropi Kale Juice

INGREDIENTS

- 1 ripe banana, peeled
- ¼ fresh pineapple, skin and core removed and cut into 1-inch strips
- 4 kale leaves

PREPARATION

1. Place the ingredients in the processor and squeeze each one of them; then place the juice in the glass, serve, and enjoy.
2. Serving Size: 1 glass (approx. 8–10 oz)

Calories: 150-180
Total Fat: 0.5-1g
Saturated Fat: 0g

Cholesterol: 0mg
Sodium: 40-60mg
Total Carbohydrate: 38-42g

Dietary Fiber: 5-7g
Sugars: 24-28g
Protein: 2-3g

Antioxidant Blast

INGREDIENTS

- 1 cup blueberries
- 1 cup halved and peeled strawberries
- 2 medium beets, quartered along with the green leaves

PREPARATION

1. Place each of the ingredients in the processor and begin to squeeze them little by little.
2. Put the juice in the fridge for 30 minutes and serve cold to refresh.
3. Serving Size: 1 glass (approx. 8–10 oz)

Calories: 130-150
Total Fat: 0.5-1g
Saturated Fat: 0g

Cholesterol: 0mg
Sodium: 110-130mg
Total Carbohydrate: 31-35g

Dietary Fiber: 7-9g
Sugars: 20-23g
Protein: 3-4g

Immune Booster Juice

INGREDIENTS

- 2 oranges, quartered and rind removed for less bitterness
- 1 medium apple, cut into eighths
- A ½-inch fresh ginger piece
- ¼ lemon, peel removed to make it less bitter

PREPARATION

1. Remember to remove the peel before blending, so it will be less bitter. Proceed to process each of the ingredients.
2. Serve in a glass and enjoy. Ginger can be put on top grated.
3. Serving Size: 1 glass (approx. 8–10 oz)

Calories: 110-130
Total Fat: 0.5-1g
Saturated Fat: 0g

Cholesterol: 0mg
Sodium: 0-5mg
Total Carbohydrate: 27-30g

Dietary Fiber: 4-5g
Sugars: 20-23g
Protein: 1-2g

Not-So-Bitter Apple Juice

INGREDIENTS

- 2 sour apples, cut into eighths
- 5 kale leaves

PREPARATION

1. Place the apples and kale in the juicer and process.
2. After doing so, serve in a glass and enjoy.
3. Serving Size: 1 glass (approx. 8–10 oz)

Calories: 100-120
Total Fat: 0.5-1g
Saturated Fat: 0g

Cholesterol: 0mg
Sodium: 30-40mg
Total Carbohydrate: 26-30g

Dietary Fiber: 4-5g
Sugars: 20-24g
Protein: 1-2g

Kickstart Juice

INGREDIENTS

- 1 orange, quartered and rind removed for less bitterness
- 1 ripe banana
- 1 cup strawberries, halved and peeled
- 2 kale leaves
- 3 carrots

PREPARATION

1. Start by squeezing all the ingredients in the order you want; oranges, ripe, strawberries, carrots, and cabbage.
2. Serve and drink immediately, or let it chill for an hour and then enjoy.
3. Serving Size: 1 glass (approx. 8–10 oz)

Calories: 150-180
Total Fat: 0.5-1g
Saturated Fat: 0g

Cholesterol: 0mg
Sodium: 80-100mg
Total Carbohydrate: 35-40g

Dietary Fiber: 7-9g
Sugars: 21-25g
Protein: 3-4g

Refreshing Cucumber Juice

INGREDIENTS

- ½ cucumber, sliced
- ¼ lemon, rind removed to reduce bitterness
- ¼ ripe cantaloupe, seeded, cut into chunks (no peeling necessary)
- 2 celery stalks

PREPARATION

1. Place all the ingredients in the juicer and process them.
2. After this, serve and enjoy.
3. Serving Size: 1 glass (approx. 8–10 oz)

Calories: 70-90
Total Fat: 0.5-1g
Saturated Fat: 0g

Cholesterol: 0mg
Sodium: 70-90mg
Total Carbohydrate: 17-20g

Dietary Fiber: 3-4g
Sugars: 12-15g
Protein: 2-3g

Cleansing Recipe

INGREDIENTS

- ¼–½ cup parsley leaves
- ½ lemon
- A 1/2-inch ginger piece
- 2 medium apples
- 2 large cucumbers
- 2 cups baby spinach leaves (or 4–6 kale leaves)
- 6 celery sticks

PREPARATION

1. Wash, prepare, and chop the products.
2. Add the items to the juicer one at a time.
3. Add ice to serve cold. You can put it in tightly closed jars or glasses in the refrigerator for 7 to 10 days. Shake it before drinking.
4. Serving Size: 1 glass (approx. 8–10 oz)

Calories: 120-150
Total Fat: 0.5-1g
Saturated Fat: 0g

Cholesterol: 0mg
Sodium: 130-160mg
Total Carbohydrate: 30-35g

Dietary Fiber: 6-8g
Sugars: 20-25g
Protein: 4-5g

Powerful Detox Juice

INGREDIENTS

- ½ lemon
- A 1/2-inch ginger
- 2 medium apples
- 2–3 medium beets
- 6 carrots

PREPARATION

1. Peel each of the foods and cut them into squares, wash them, and leave them ready.
2. Place each of them in the juicer one at a time.
3. Serve cold over ice. If you keep it sealed, you can leave it for up to a week in the refrigerator.
4. Serving Size: 1 glass (approx. 8-10 oz)

Calories: 180-220
Total Fat: 0.5-1g
Saturated Fat: 0g

Cholesterol: 0mg
Sodium: 180-220mg
Total Carbohydrate: 45-50g

Dietary Fiber: 8-10g
Sugars: 30-35g
Protein: 4-5g

Sweet Carrot to Clean and Reinforce

INGREDIENTS

- ¼ cup parsley (optional)
- 10 large carrots
- 2 medium apples

PREPARATION

1. Clean and peel each of the foods.
2. Put them in the juicer each one at a time.
3. Serve cold over ice. You can keep it in the refrigerator for up to a week, and you can drink it cold or at room temperature.
4. Serving Size: 1 glass (approx. 8-10 oz)

Calories: 170-200
Total Fat: 0.5-1g
Saturated Fat: 0g

Cholesterol: 0mg
Sodium: 180-220mg
Total Carbohydrate: 40-45g

Dietary Fiber: 8-10g
Sugars: 30-35g
Protein: 2-3g

Naturally Sweet Green Detox Juice

In this green juice, the spinach is smooth, the parsley is refreshing, lemon and ginger energize, and cucumbers add mineral-rich water. Apples are naturally sweet, so we don't add any extra sugar or fruit except lemon. If you find the juice too tart, consider adding a few carrots or an extra apple to the juicer. If you are sensitive to the spiciness of ginger, add a small amount first, then add more.

INGREDIENTS

- 1 medium lemon
- 1 medium green apple, rinsed and cored
- 1 large seedless cucumber (hothouse or English), rinsed
- 2 cups packed baby spinach leaves
- A 1-inch-long fresh ginger piece, well scrubbed
- A handful of parsley leaves and stems

PREPARATION

1. Vegetables:
2. Chop the apple, cucumber, and ginger into small-enough pieces to fit easily through the juicer.
3. Cut the yellow rind off the lemon, leaving only the white pith and pulp of the lemon. Cut it into slices and remove the seeds.
4. Process of making the juice:
5. Reserve about half of the lemon. Start the juicer and push everything, alternating between the vegetables and the cucumber, apple, and lemon more firmly.
6. When everything but the lemon you set aside has been squeezed, stir it all up and confirm the acidity.
7. Add the remaining lemon if you think you can tolerate it. Or if the juice is very sour, you can add a couple of washed unpeeled carrots or another apple without a core.
8. Serving Size: 1 glass (approx. 8–10 oz)

Calories: 90-110
Total Fat: 0.5-1g
Saturated Fat: 0g

Cholesterol: 0mg
Sodium: 40-60mg
Total Carbohydrate: 20-25g

Dietary Fiber: 4-5g
Sugars: 13-15g
Protein: 2-3g

Kale Detox Juice

INGREDIENTS

- 1 ½ oz lemon juice (about 1 lemon)
- 2 oz cucumber juice (about ¼ large cucumber)
- 5 oz kale juice (about 1 bunch of kale)
- 5 oz Fuji apple juice (about 2 apples)

PREPARATION

1. Squeeze the ingredients in the processor and put and place each one in a separate glass.
2. Measure 5 oz kale juice, 5 oz fuji apple juice, 2 oz cucumber juice, and 1 ½ oz lemon juice.
3. Mix before serving. You can also seal and store it in the fridge.
4. Serving Size: 1 glass (approx. 8-10 oz)

Calories: 100-120
Total Fat: 0.5-1g
Saturated Fat: 0g

Cholesterol: 0mg
Sodium: 40-60mg
Total Carbohydrate: 25-30g

Dietary Fiber: 3-4g
Sugars: 18-20g
Protein: 2-3g

Pineapple and Ginger Cleansing Juice

INGREDIENTS

- 1 lime, peeled
- A 2-inch fresh ginger root, peeled
- 3 turmeric pieces
- 3 cups fresh pineapple, peeled

PREPARATION

1. Chop and peel the pineapple, ginger, turmeric, and lime.
2. Place the pineapple, ginger, turmeric, and lime one at a time in your juicer to process.
3. Before serving, stir the juice with a wooden spoon to combine well.
4. Pour in ¼ full glass of juice and ¼ full glass of crushed ice, and top up the rest of the glass with coconut water or distilled water. You can garnish it with lime slices and fresh mint.
5. Serving Size: 1 glass (approx. 8-10 oz)

Calories: 150-180
Total Fat: 0.5-1g
Saturated Fat: 0g

Cholesterol: 0mg
Sodium: 5-10mg
Total Carbohydrate: 40-45g

Dietary Fiber: 3-4g
Sugars: 30-35g
Protein: 1-2g

Carrot Juice With Orange and Ginger

INGREDIENTS

- 2 peeled and clean carrots
- 2 peeled oranges, only with the white
- 1 peeled, lemon only with the white
- A small piece of ginger to grate

PREPARATION

1. Wash each item of food, including whole carrots. Cut into pieces small enough to fit through the feed tube of your juicer.
2. Place the pieces of fruit and vegetables in the tube of the juicer or the model that you handle.
3. Combine hard and soft pieces of fruits and vegetables to get the most juice out of fruits and vegetables.
4. Serve the glass of carrot juice immediately. It is best to serve right after making it.
5. Serving Size: 1 glass (approx. 8–10 oz)

Calories: 120-140
Total Fat: 0.5-1g
Saturated Fat: 0g

Cholesterol: 0mg
Sodium: 30-50mg
Total Carbohydrate: 30-35g

Dietary Fiber: 4-5g
Sugars: 20-25g
Protein: 2-3g

Detox Beetroot Juice

INGREDIENTS

- 1 beetroot
- 2 carrots
- 2 celery ribs
- 1 lemon
- 1 cucumber
- 2 green and red apples
- 1 bunch of flat-leaf parsley

PREPARATION

1. Wash everything and chop it into smaller pieces so that you can put them in the juicer tube.
2. Put each piece in the juicer, then serve immediately or chill first in the fridge.
3. Serving Size: 1 glass (approx. 8-10 oz)

Calories: 150-180
Total Fat: 1-2g
Saturated Fat: 0g

Cholesterol: 0mg
Sodium: 100-150mg
Total Carbohydrate: 35-40g

Dietary Fiber: 6-8g
Sugars: 25-30g
Protein: 2-3g

Green Vegetable Detox Juice

INGREDIENTS

- 1 lime or lemon, skin removed
- 1 bunch of flat-leaf parsley
- 1 green apple
- 1 English cucumber
- 3 kale leaves or 1 handful of baby spinach
- 8 celery stalks (about 1 celery head)

PREPARATION

1. Chop and wash the vegetables so they can easily enter the juicer.
2. Place the vegetables through the tube, combining hard and soft textured ones to make the juicing process easy.
3. Enjoy it right away or put leftovers in a tightly sealed container in the fridge.
4. Serving Size: 1 glass (approx. 8-10 oz)

Calories: 70-100
Total Fat: 0-1g
Saturated Fat: 0g

Cholesterol: 0mg
Sodium: 100-150mg
Total Carbohydrate: 16-20g

Dietary Fiber: 4-6g
Sugars: 9-12g
Protein: 2-3g

Anti-Inflammatory Juice

INGREDIENTS

- ½ green apple
- ½ cucumber
- 1 cup spinach
- 1 cup pineapple
- 1 lemon
- 1 ginger nut
- 4 celery stalks

PREPARATION

1. Place all the ingredients in the vegetable juicer.
2. Gently stir the juice and drink immediately.
3. Serving Size: 1 glass (approx. 8-10 oz)

Calories: 80-100
Total Fat: 0-1g
Saturated Fat: 0g

Cholesterol: 0mg
Sodium: 60-80mg
Total Carbohydrate: 20-25g

Dietary Fiber: 4-6g
Sugars: 12-15g
Protein: 2-3g

Detox Ginger Shot

This is a recipe that has ginger and turmeric juice, and it intensely helps you to work the natural immune system at home. It is rich in vitamins, minerals, and antioxidants, boosts the immune system, helps give you energy, and is an excellent cold killer, in addition to working your body to cleanse it of bad energy.

INGREDIENTS

- 1 tsp turmeric
- 1 apple
- 2 lemons
- 3 tbsp agave syrup
- 3 ½ oz (100 g) ginger
- 4 tangerines (mandarins)
- Approx. ⅔ cup (150 ml) water or fruit juice
- A pinch of black pepper (optional)
- Tip: If the juice gets spicy due to the slices of ginger and turmeric, you can put an apple on it. Other fruits like oranges, grapes, pineapples, pears, etc. are also a great vitamin-rich addition!

PREPARATION

1. First, start by washing the ginger and coarsely chop it. Completely remove the peel from the lemons and tangerines and chop the fruit into large pieces.
2. Wash and core the apple and also cut it into large pieces.
3. Then simply put all the ingredients in the juicer one by one and go placing them in a container.
4. When finished, combine the entire mixture by hand.
5. After that, place the energy drink in a sealable bottle or several small bottles. You can keep them in the fridge for about a week, and they can also be frozen.
6. Serving Size: 1 shot (approx. 2-3 oz)

Calories: 60-80
Total Fat: 0-1g
Saturated Fat: 0g

Cholesterol: 0mg
Sodium: 0-10mg
Total Carbohydrate: 15-20g

Dietary Fiber: 1-2g
Sugars: 10-15g
Protein: 1-2g

Citrus Season Elixir

INGREDIENTS

- 1 tbsp fresh ginger
- 1 lemon
- 1 large red grapefruit
- 2 apples
- 2 blood oranges
- 5 carrots

PREPARATION

1. Start with refrigerated foods if you have them. Chop all ingredients into 1-inch pieces.
2. Put the ingredients one at a time in the juicer working in a slow mode. Start with an ingredient that isn't as juicy (like ginger) and combine it with an ingredient that makes a lot of juice (like carrots). This ensures that the juicy ingredients get rid of the not-so-juicy ingredients through the juicer and you get more in your cup!
3. After you manage to squeeze all the ingredients, stir the juice and pour it into glasses.
4. Optionally (but elegant and fun!): Add a blood orange to garnish each glass and enjoy!
5. Serving Size: 1 glass (approximately 8-10 oz)

Calories: 120-150
Total Fat: 0-1g
Saturated Fat: 0g

Cholesterol: 0mg
Sodium: 50-100mg
Total Carbohydrate: 30-40g

Dietary Fiber: 4-6g
Sugars: 20-25g
Protein: 2-3g

Celery and Cucumber Recipe

INGREDIENTS

- A 1½-inch fresh ginger nut, without skin
- 1 celery head, cut into stalks
- 1 lime, skin cut
- 1 apple, red or green, sliced
- 5 small Persian cucumbers, washed with the tips trimmed

PREPARATION

1. Place all the ingredients in the juicer, alternating the hard and soft pieces.
2. Serve immediately.
3. Serving Size: 1 glass (approximately 8-10 oz)

Calories: 70-80
Total Fat: 0.5-1g
Saturated Fat: 0g

Cholesterol: 0mg
Sodium: 80-100mg
Total Carbohydrate: 16-18g

Dietary Fiber: 3-4g
Sugars: 10-12g
Protein: 1-2g

Orange, Carrot, Mango, and Turmeric Juice

A refreshing tropical juice of carrot, mango, orange, and turmeric. This powerful immune-boosting juice tastes like sunshine in a bottle.

INGREDIENTS

- 1 ½ cups water
- A 1-inch turmeric root piece, peeled (or use about 1 tsp turmeric powder)
- 1 mango, peeled and cored
- 1 orange, peeled
- 1/8 tsp black pepper (for turmeric absorption)
- 3 large carrots, peeled

PREPARATION

1. Wash and dry each of the foods. Remove the skins. If you won't strain it, be careful to peel the carrots or they will leave a gritty texture.
2. Put all the ingredients in the juicer and combine everything after you process it in the equipment.
3. Optional: Strain the juice using a bag of walnut milk so that it has a very smooth finish without pulp. Enjoy!
4. Serving Size: 1 glass (approximately 8–10 oz)

Calories: 150-180
Total Fat: 0-1g
Saturated Fat: 0g

Cholesterol: 0mg
Sodium: 60-80mg
Total Carbohydrate: 35-40g

Dietary Fiber: 5-6g
Sugars: 25-30g
Protein: 2-3g

Celyne's Green Juice

INGREDIENTS

- 1 kale leaf
- 1 lemon, peeled
- 1 green apple, quartered
- 1 cup fresh spinach
- 2 oranges, peeled

PREPARATION

1. Process the oranges with the lemon, green apple, spinach, and kale until the juice comes out.
2. Serve cold or fresh as you prefer.
3. Serving Size: 1 glass (approximately 8–10 oz)

Calories: 100-120
Total Fat: 0-1g
Saturated Fat: 0g

Cholesterol: 0mg
Sodium: 30-50mg
Total Carbohydrate: 25-30g

Dietary Fiber: 5-7g
Sugars: 15-20g
Protein: 2-3g

Aloe Vera Juice

INGREDIENTS

- 1 cup water
- 1 large lemon
- 2 tbsp edible aloe gel, or cut from whole aloe leaves without peel and latex
- 2 medium cucumbers
- A 1-inch ginger piece, peeled

PREPARATION

1. Wash and dry the food. Cut the tip off the cucumbers, then quarter them to fit into the juicer. Cut the lemon in half. Peel the ginger.
2. Squeeze the lemon juice. Put the cucumbers and ginger in the juicer. Process each of the foods and leave a single mixture, add water to it.
3. Strain the liquid through a cheesecloth or nut milk bag and squeeze to get all the juice out. Discard the excess pulp if you want, although you can save the pulp for one of the recipes at the end.
4. Cut the thorns on the sides of the aloe leaf. Cut a face out of the aloe leaf so that you have access to the gel. Scoop out 2 tablespoons of the clear aloe gel, taking care of the yellow-tinted gel closest to the leaf surface.
5. Put the aloe gel in the juicer. Combine in a setting for you to process and add to the liquid.
6. Pour the juice over some ice and enjoy!
7. Serving Size: 1 glass (approximately 8-10 oz)

Calories: 50-70
Total Fat: 0g
Saturated Fat: 0g

Cholesterol: 0mg
Sodium: 10-20mg
Total Carbohydrate: 12-15g

Dietary Fiber: 2-3g
Sugars: 6-8g
Protein: 1-2g

Celery and Lemon Juice

INGREDIENTS

- 1 lime, peeled (optional, for better flavor)
- 2 bunches of celery

PREPARATION

1. Prepare the celery for juicing by cutting the bottom and top of the stalks from the two bunches.
2. Place the celery stalks in a colander in the sink. Wash the celery and let it dry.
3. Process the celery and lime in the juicer.
4. Serve the juice immediately or place the leftovers in an airtight jar in the refrigerator. You can take it within 3 days after juicing.
5. Serving Size: 1 glass (approximately 8-10 oz)

Calories: 30-40
Total Fat: 0g
Saturated Fat: 0g

Cholesterol: 0mg
Sodium: 100-200mg
Total Carbohydrate: 6-8g

Dietary Fiber: 2-3g
Sugars: 3-4g
Protein: 1-2g

Cabbage and Apple Juice

INGREDIENTS

- ½ lemon, peeled
- 1 cucumber
- 1 piece (1 inch) fresh ginger
- 2 green apples, halved
- 4 celery stalks, without leaves
- 6 kale leaves

PREPARATION

1. Gather all the ingredients.
2. Process the kale, celery, cucumber, green apples, lemon, and ginger in a juicer.
3. Serve immediately or refrigerate in a glass jar for up to a day; shake before drinking.
4. Serving Size: 1 glass (approximately 8-10 oz)

Calories: 100-120
Total Fat: 0.5-1g
Saturated Fat: 0g

Cholesterol: 0mg
Sodium: 80-100mg
Total Carbohydrate: 25-30g

Dietary Fiber: 5-7g
Sugars: 18-20g
Protein: 2-3g

Zinger Juice

INGREDIENTS

- 2 lemons, peeled, seeded, and quartered
- 2 apples, quartered
- 2 beets, sliced and chopped
- 2 carrots, chopped

PREPARATION

1. Press the lemons, carrots, apples, and beets in the juicer and into a large glass.
2. Seek to leave the carrots and apples with the peel, since a good part of the nutrients are in the peel. They also give fiber to the juice. This juice is packed with beta-carotene, which is great for the skin, eyes, cells, and the release of toxins from the body.
3. Serving Size: 1 glass (approximately 8–10 oz)

Calories: 150-180
Total Fat: 1-2g
Saturated Fat: 0g

Cholesterol: 0mg
Sodium: 100-120mg
Total Carbohydrate: 35-40g

Dietary Fiber: 7-9g
Sugars: 25-30g
Protein: 2-3g

Mango and Banana Juice

INGREDIENTS

- ½ lemon, peeled
- ½ orange, peeled
- 1 mango, peeled, seeded, and cut into wedges
- 1 banana, peeled
- 2 apples, cut into chunks
- 2 slices of fresh ginger root

PREPARATION

1. Process the banana, along with the lemon, mango, orange, apples, and ginger in the juicer.
2. Serving Size: 1 glass (approximately 8–10 oz)

Calories: 200-250
Total Fat: 0-1g
Saturated Fat: 0g

Cholesterol: 0mg
Sodium: 0-5mg
Total Carbohydrate: 50-60g

Dietary Fiber: 5-7g
Sugars: 35-45g
Protein: 1-2g

Citrus Juice, Turmeric, and Ginger

INGREDIENTS

- ½ tsp ground turmeric
- ½ peeled lemon
- 1 orange, peeled and cut
- 1 piece (1 inch) fresh ginger
- 2 Fuji apples, cored and sliced

PREPARATION

1. Process the apples, the orange, the lemon, and the ginger in a juicer; stir in turmeric until evenly incorporated.
2. Serving Size: 1 glass (approximately 8–10 oz)

Calories: 150-200
Total Fat: 1-2g
Saturated Fat: 0g

Cholesterol: 0mg
Sodium: 5-10mg
Total Carbohydrate: 35-40g

Dietary Fiber: 5-7g
Sugars: 25-30g
Protein: 1-2g

Zinger Orange

INGREDIENTS

- A ½-inch fresh ginger root piece
- 1 lb carrots, washed and cut
- 2 oranges, peeled

PREPARATION

1. Prepare ginger, carrot, and orange juice by combining everything in the juicer.
2. Serve immediately.

Calories: 120-140
Total Fat: 0.5-1g
Saturated Fat: 0g

Cholesterol: 0mg
Sodium: 70-90mg
Total Carbohydrate: 28-32g

Dietary Fiber: 5-7g
Sugars: 18-22g
Protein: 2-3g

Rainbow Juice

INGREDIENTS

- ¼ cup fresh blueberries, or more to taste
- 1 piece (1 inch) fresh ginger, peeled
- 1 cup of fresh spinach
- 2 small beets, peeled
- 2 oranges, peeled
- 2 carrots

PREPARATION

1. Put carrots, spinach, beets, oranges, cranberries, and ginger through a juicer to create a juice that you serve and enjoy.

Calories: 150-180
Total Fat: 0.5-1g
Saturated Fat: 0g

Cholesterol: 0mg
Sodium: 100-120mg
Total Carbohydrate: 35-40g

Dietary Fiber: 7-9g
Sugars: 25-30g
Protein: 3-4g

Spiced Carrot and Sweet Potato Juice of Life

INGREDIENTS

- ¼ tsp ground cinnamon
- 1 (1-inch) piece fresh ginger root, peeled
- 1 pinch of ground nutmeg
- 3 large peeled sweet potatoes
- 3 large carrots

PREPARATION

1. Process the sweet potatoes, carrots, and ginger in the juicer, arranging them from hardest to softest.
2. Stir the ground cinnamon and nutmeg into the juice.
3. Serving Size: 1 glass (approximately 8–10 oz)

Calories: 200-250
Total Fat: 0.5-1g
Saturated Fat: 0g

Cholesterol: 0mg
Sodium: 100-120mg
Total Carbohydrate: 45-50g

Dietary Fiber: 8-10g
Sugars: 12-15g
Protein: 3-4g

Immunity Juice Boost

INGREDIENTS

- 1 (2-inch) piece fresh ginger root
- 3 large navy oranges, peeled
- Ice cubes
- 2 (1 ½-inch) fresh turmeric pieces

PREPARATION

1. Process the ginger, turmeric, and oranges in a juicer in the order listed.
2. Pour over ice and drink immediately.
3. Notes: This recipe can make 12 to 16 fluid ounces, however, it will depend on the oranges.
4. A 2-inch piece of ginger weighs about 1 oz. 2 (1 1/2-inch) pieces of turmeric weigh about 1/2 oz. You don't need to peel ginger or turmeric, but turmeric does stain, so handle it carefully. For a spicier flavor, put more ginger in it.
5. The juice from a centrifugal juicer must be consumed within 24 hours. The juice made with a masticating juicer (cold pressed) should be taken within 48 hours.

Calories: 120-150
Total Fat: 0-1g
Saturated Fat: 0g

Cholesterol: 0mg
Sodium: 10-20mg
Total Carbohydrate: 30-35g

Dietary Fiber: 5-7g
Sugars: 20-25g
Protein: 2-3g

Green Dragon Juice

INGREDIENTS

- ¼ large lemon
- ⅓ small jalapeno pepper
- 1 pinch of salt
- 1 cup fresh spinach, or to taste
- 1 cup ice, or to taste
- 1 tomato, quartered
- 2 sprigs of fresh parsley, or more to taste
- 2 celery stalks

PREPARATION

1. Process the spinach, lemon, parsley, celery, jalapeño pepper, and tomato through a juice extractor. Add salt to season the juice.
2. Put ice in the glass and place the juice.
3. Notes: Adjust the lemons to your taste. If the lemon is small, use half; if it's larger, use a quarter or a third. There is no need to peel the lemons.
4. Since the heat of jalapeños can vary widely, start with 1/4 to 1/3 of a small pepper and adjust accordingly.
5. Serving Size: 1 glass (approximately 8–10 oz)

Calories: 30-40
Total Fat: 0.5-1g
Saturated Fat: 0g

Cholesterol: 0mg
Sodium: 80-100mg
Total Carbohydrate: 6-8g

Dietary Fiber: 2-3g
Sugars: 3-4g
Protein: 1-2g

Clean Green Juice

INGREDIENTS

- 1 tbsp water, or as needed
- 1 tbsp freshly squeezed lemon juice
- 1 cucumber, coarsely chopped
- Granny Smith apples, halved and cored
- 3 Romaine lettuce leaves
- 3 kale leaves
- 5 fresh parsley sprigs
- 5 celery stalks, without leaves

PREPARATION

1. Place the apples, cucumber, kale, celery, Romaine lettuce leaves, parsley, lemon juice, and water in a blender or juicer.
2. Process until you reach the desired consistency. Add more water as needed.
3. Serving Size: 1 glass (approximately 8–10 oz)

Calories: 80-100
Total Fat: 0-1g
Saturated Fat: 0g

Cholesterol: 0mg
Sodium: 50-100mg
Total Carbohydrate: 20-25g

Dietary Fiber: 4-6g
Sugars: 12-15g
Protein: 2-3g

CHAPTER 6
ANTI-AGING AND SKIN BRIGHTENING JUICE RECIPES

After seeing the recipes to detoxify the body, it is time to see how to recover the glow of the skin and take anti-aging juices; these recipes are quick to make and very effective.

When it comes to slowing down or reducing the effects of aging, any strategy of natural origin will interest and benefit us.

We are talking about recipes we can prepare every day to provide us with all the treasures of anti-oxidants, hydration, and vitamin C, in addition to improving our general health. Therefore, they are ideal for smoothing wrinkles or restoring the elasticity of our skin.

We all know that there are no miracles in aging. There are methods, treatments, and above all, the inescapable assumption that the passage of time is inevitable.

Now, as the years go by, it's always fun to be active. Our main purpose will be to take care of ourselves, feel good, and pay maximum attention to what we eat.

Today in our space we propose the following recommendations to drink one or more of the following natural juices daily. They are very healthy and will help you reduce the footprint of the passage of time. Pay attention!

Homemade Citrus Juice

INGREDIENTS

- ¼ lime
- ½ lemon
- 1 grapefruit
- 10 tangerines
- 5 oranges
- Agave syrup to taste (optional)

PREPARATION

1. Rinse the fruits under running water. Peel the tangerines, oranges, and grapefruit. Process them in the juicer. Squeeze the lemon and lime.
2. Taste it and sweeten it with agave syrup if you feel it necessary!
3. Serving Size: 1 cup (240 ml) of citrus juice

Calories: 100-120 calories
Total Fat: 0 grams
Saturated Fat: 0 grams

Cholesterol: 0 milligrams
Sodium: 0-5 milligrams
Total Carbohydrate: 25-30 grams

Dietary Fiber: 2-4 grams
Sugars: 18-24 grams
Protein: 2-3 grams

Spinach, Celery, and Lemon Green Juice

INGREDIENTS

- ½ tbsp freshly squeezed lemon juice
- 1 cup water
- 1 cup ice
- 1/2 cucumber, peeled and coarsely chopped
- 2 celery ribs, chopped
- 2 medium apples, cut into chunks
- 3 cups baby spinach leaves (or chopped baby spinach or kale)
- Optional: a 1/2-inch piece of ginger, peeled

PREPARATION

1. Wash each of the foods.
2. Place the spinach, apples, celery, cucumber, and lemon juice in the processor in the juicer. Squeeze, then put water until smooth.
3. Pass the mixture through a fine or medium-mesh strainer or a nut milk bag into a mug (medium mesh leaves much of the fiber in the juice; fine mesh leaves it completely clear). Place it in a glass and serve, or leave refrigerated until serving time.
4. Serving Size: Approximately 1 glass (8-10 oz)

Calories: 70-90 kcal
Total Fat: 0.5-1g
Saturated Fat: 0g

Cholesterol: 0mg
Sodium: 60-80mg
Total Carbohydrate: 18-22g

Dietary Fiber: 4-6g
Sugars: 11-14g
Protein: 2-3g

Broccoli, Cucumber, and Lemon Juice

INGREDIENTS

- 2 broccoli florets
- 1 cucumber
- 1 lemon

PREPARATION

1. The first thing for this recipe is that you place all the ingredients in the juicer.
2. Add the broccoli florets, cucumber, and squeezed lemon juice and combine until smooth.
3. Add the juice to a glass and make sure to drink it right away so that you get the most benefits from the nutrients.
4. You can drink this juice fresh, but you can also leave it in the refrigerator for up to a day.
5. Serving Size: Approximately 1 glass (8-10 oz)

Calories: 40-60 kcal
Total Fat: 0.5-1g
Saturated Fat: 0g

Cholesterol: 0mg
Sodium: 20-30mg
Total Carbohydrate: 10-15g

Dietary Fiber: 3-4g
Sugars: 3-5g
Protein: 2-3g

Beet Juice With Apple

INGREDIENTS

- A ½-inch ginger piece, peeled
- ½ lemon or lime
- 2 carrots
- 2 celery stalks
- 1 big apple
- 1 small beet

PREPARATION

1. Start by washing all the vegetables and fruits under running water and drying them.
2. Cut and peel the beetroot into long slices. Chop the apple into long pieces and remove the core. Cut and peel both the carrot and the celery into long pieces.
3. Put a glass or container under your juicer and turn it on.
4. Process each of the ingredients (carrot, beetroot, apple, celery, ginger), except the lemon, alternately through a juicer.
5. Squeeze half a lemon into the prepared juice and combine well. Pour into a chilled serving glass and serve. Drink immediately.
6. **Tips and variations:**
7. Choose firm and small beets. Also, we put sweetened apples in it, but you can use them with any type of apple you choose.
8. Pure beet juice is very strong, always combine it with some other fruit or vegetable juice to avoid possible side effects.
9. If you use organic vegetables and fruits, do not peel them.
10. Serving Size: Approximately 1 glass (8-10 oz)

Calories: 120-140 kcal
Total Fat: 0.5-1g
Saturated Fat: 0g

Cholesterol: 0mg
Sodium: 130-150mg
Total Carbohydrate: 30-35g

Dietary Fiber: 6-8g
Sugars: 20-24g
Protein: 2-3g

Cilantro Lemonade With Honey

I can certainly say that this green juice is very delicious. This cilantro lemonade is excellent and I dare you to try it! Also, this is a green lemonade recipe you can make in no time with the juicer.

INGREDIENTS

- 1 large bunch of cilantro, 3 cups, chopped (if the bunches are small, use 2!)
- 1−3 tbsp honey or maple syrup, or to taste
- ½ cup fresh lemon juice (3−4 juicy lemons)
- 2 ½ cups water
- ¼ tsp salt

PREPARATION

1. Wash the coriander and chop it into large pieces.
2. Squeeze the lemons in the processor.
3. Add the missing ingredients and mix.
4. Pass it through a strainer to catch any pulp and serve!
5. Notes: If you want a thinner consistency, don't need to sift.
6. Alternatively, you can use a juicer to squeeze the cilantro and lemon juice. However, liquid sweeteners are easier to mix.
7. This will store well in the fridge for 2 days but is best eaten the day it's made.
8. Serving Size: Approximately 1 glass (8-10 oz)

Calories: 80-100 kcal
Total Fat: 0-0.5g
Saturated Fat: 0g

Cholesterol: 0mg
Sodium: 160-200mg
Total Carbohydrate: 21-25g

Dietary Fiber: 1-2g
Sugars: 15-18g
Protein: 1-2g

Cucumber, Celery, and Green Apple Juice

INGREDIENTS

- ½ broccoli head
- ½ green apple
- ¾−1 cucumber (depending on size)
- 1 whole fennel bulb (if you don't have fennel, use a bunch of Swiss chard and a handful of parsley
- 6 celery pieces

PREPARATION

1. Take the slices of green apple and fennel (or Swiss chard if substituting)
2. Squeeze both vegetables and fruits through a juicer and into a cup.
3. Enjoy with ice or as is.
4. The good thing is that you can squeeze a little juice from a lemon on top.
5. Serving Size: Approximately 1 glass (8-10 oz)

Calories: 40-60 kcal
Total Fat: 0.5-1g
Saturated Fat: 0g

Cholesterol: 0mg
Sodium: 50-70mg
Total Carbohydrate: 10-15g

Dietary Fiber: 3-4g
Sugars: 5-7g
Protein: 2-3g

Green Juice With Ingredients for the Skin

Green juice is an excellent way to introduce vegetables into our body that we normally don't eat much, just like other similar recipes that I have taught you. One thing I love about juicing is that adding your favorite fruit, like an apple, to the mix will turn your juice into a delicious drink, even with vegetables you don't like very much! You can barely taste the vegetables! Best of all, it doesn't get any fresher and healthier than this!

The health benefits depend on the ratio of the ingredients, but most green juices are rich in vitamins, antioxidants, and chlorophyll to help detoxify your body.

INGREDIENTS

- 2 kale leaves
- 4 large apples
- 6 celery stalks

PREPARATION

1. Pass each of the ingredients under running water.
2. Scoop out the core of the apples. Remove ends from kale leaves. Put them in a juicer along with the celery stalks, which you will cut into smaller pieces.
3. The juice will take 1 or 2 minutes to make.
4. Once the juice is made, put it in glasses and serve immediately.
5. Serving Size: Approximately 1 glass (8-10 oz)

Calories: 100-120 kcal
Total Fat: 0-0.5g
Saturated Fat: 0g

Cholesterol: 0mg
Sodium: 30-40mg
Total Carbohydrate: 27-30g

Dietary Fiber: 4-5g
Sugars: 20-22g
Protein: 1-2g

Broccoli, Pear, and Ginger Juice

INGREDIENTS

- 1 pear
- 2 broccoli florets
- 1 inch of ginger

PREPARATION

1. Place all the ingredients into the juicer and blend until smooth.
2. After processing it, serve and enjoy it.
3. You can store the leftover juice in the refrigerator for a day.
4. Serving Size: Approximately 1 glass (8-10 oz)

Calories: 60-80 kcal
Total Fat: 0.5-1g
Saturated Fat: 0g

Cholesterol: 0mg
Sodium: 30-50mg
Total Carbohydrate: 15-20g

Dietary Fiber: 3-4g
Sugars: 9-12g
Protein: 2-3g

Kale Juice

- 2 lemons
- 6 celery stalks
- 1 (2-inch) ginger nut
- 1 apple, cut in two
- 2 cucumbers

1. Wash and dry the ingredients. Take this to the juicer. Start with the kale, then add the ginger, celery, lemon, and cucumber, or do it in any order you like. Place the apple last so you remove any rest of the other ingredients.
2. Drink immediately or place in airtight glass bottles, Mason jars, or a pitcher to refrigerate and drink within 72 hours. Don't freeze it.
3. You can store this juice in airtight glass bottles for up to 3 days in the refrigerator. This way you can get the most out of the vitamins and nutrients before the juice goes rancid.
4. Serving Size: Approximately 1 glass (8-10 oz)

Calories: 80-100 kcal
Total Fat: 0.5-1g
Saturated Fat: 0g

Cholesterol: 0mg
Sodium: 60-80mg
Total Carbohydrate: 20-25g

Dietary Fiber: 3-4g
Sugars: 12-15g
Protein: 2-3g

Carrot, Dates, and Beetroot Juice

Do you use beets for brighter cheeks? Now you can use it to reveal glowing skin from within. Carrot and beetroot go together perfectly, one of the best elixirs nature has to offer. Beetroot is rich in essential nutrients such as potassium, iron, zinc, folic acid, manganese, and vitamin C. These nutrients are reputed to be the gift of purifying the blood and helping to reveal healthy skin.

Carrots are rich in vitamin A, which fights acne, wrinkles, fine lines, and hyperpigmentation problems. It is rich in fiber, which is good for bowel movement and excretion, thus cleaning the stomach. Now who wants to run home and make this juice?

- 1 carrot
- 3 dates, without the seeds
- ½ beetroot

1. Cut the carrot and beetroot into pieces and put them together with the dates in the juicer.
2. Add 2-3 tablespoons of water and mix well until you get a very runny appearance.
3. Serving Size: Approximately 1 glass (8-10 oz)

Calories: 130-150 kcal
Total Fat: 0.5-1g
Saturated Fat: 0g

Cholesterol: 0mg
Sodium: 70-100mg
Total Carbohydrate: 30-35g

Dietary Fiber: 4-5g
Sugars: 23-25g
Protein: 2-3g

Tomato and Carrot Juice

Ripe red tomatoes can do wonders to change your skin. This superfood juice helps reduce break-outs, clear blemishes, and even out skin tone, as well as reverse the signs of aging. This is an effective summer drink to help cool down the body. It contains an antioxidant called lycopene, which is a natural sunscreen that protects the skin from within. You should know that carrots are good for the eyes and great for skin problems. They contain Vitamin A to help fight acne, wrinkles, hyperpigmentation, and uneven skin tone. It is also rich in fiber, which helps to cleanse the stomach and improve facial glow. It is also a rich source of vitamin C and potassium, which help improve skin elasticity and new cell production. Drinking this juice daily is good for your health.

INGREDIENTS

- 1 tbsp flax seeds
- 1 carrot
- 2 tomatoes

PREPARATION

1. Cut the tomato and carrot into pieces and take them to the juicer with the flax seeds.
2. Mix well so that you create a runny consistency.
3. Serving Size: Approximately 1 glass (8–10 oz)

Calories: 70-80 kcal
Total Fat: 2-3g
Saturated Fat: 0.2-0.3g

Cholesterol: 0mg
Sodium: 40-50mg
Total Carbohydrate: 15-18g

Dietary Fiber: 4-5g
Sugars: 7-9g
Protein: 2-3g

Papaya Juice

Papaya is a wonderful vegetable with many health benefits. We all know of its use in beauty products to reveal brighter and clearer skin. Did you know that you can achieve hyperpigmentation results even faster if you drink this miracle botanical drink? Its sap contains an enzyme called papain that removes impurities from the skin, leaving it looking clear and luminous. The papaya is smooth and tender, easy to mix, and melts in your mouth. Drinking papaya juice regularly can make the skin smooth, healthy, and radiant as it works well to remove toxins from within.

INGREDIENTS

- 1 tbsp flax seeds
- 1 ripe papaya

PREPARATION

1. Cut the papaya into pieces and put them in the juicer with the flax seeds. Combine well so that you get a liquid consistency.
2. Serving Size: Approximately 1 glass (8–10 oz)

Calories: 90-100 kcal
Total Fat: 2-3g
Saturated Fat: 0.2-0.3g

Cholesterol: 0mg
Sodium: 10-15mg
Total Carbohydrate: 20-25g

Dietary Fiber: 5-6g
Sugars: 12-15g
Protein: 1-2g

Cucumber Mint Juice

Mint is synonymous with achieving a greater sense of vitality and refreshing your mood. But did you know that it not only tastes good but is also excellent for taking care of your skin? Mint has active antibacterial qualities and salicylic acid, which prevents the appearance of acne.

It also has vitamin A which controls acne problems and breakouts. Cucumbers, on the other hand, do not affect your stomach and help you stay hydrated. It has a high moisture content which is good for the skin. It is also enriched with silica to enhance your natural complexion and add radiance. Drinking juice made from these two ingredients improves skin condition and reveals beautiful and radiant skin.

INGREDIENTS

- 1 cucumber
- 1 handful of mint leaves

PREPARATION

1. Chop the cucumber into pieces and squeeze them into the equipment with the mint leaves.
2. Mix well so that you achieve a liquid texture. If necessary, add a little water.
3. Serving Size: Approximately 1 glass (8–10 oz)

Calories: 10-15 kcal
Total Fat: 0g
Saturated Fat: 0g

Cholesterol: 0mg
Sodium: 0-5mg
Total Carbohydrate: 2-3g

Dietary Fiber: 0-1g
Sugars: 1-2g
Protein: 0-1g

Broccoli Juice

Broccoli is a fibrous vegetable, like cabbage, it is rich in vitamin C. Its juice is good for the skin. This vegetable is low in cholesterol and increases the inner glow. Broccoli contains a substance called glucoraphanin that can help repair the skin.

INGREDIENTS

- 1 broccoli
- A handful of flax seeds

PREPARATION

1. Chop the broccoli into pieces and put them in the juicer with the flax seeds.
2. Mix well to create a runny consistency. If necessary add a little water.
3. Serving Size: Approximately 1 glass (8–10 oz)

Calories: 20-30 kcal
Total Fat: 1-2g
Saturated Fat: 0g

Cholesterol: 0mg
Sodium: 10-20mg
Total Carbohydrate: 4-5g

Dietary Fiber: 1-2g
Sugars: 1-2g
Protein: 2-3g

Apple, Strawberry, and Kale Juice

Who doesn't like red fruits in smoothies? Strawberries are a rich source of elegans, folate, and vitamin C. Each ingredient has anti-inflammatory properties to help fight free radical damage. Apples are rich in vitamin A, which helps skin feel soft and smooth. Kale is a powerful leafy green that is known to do wonders for your skin. It contains vitamins A and K, which have been shown to help reduce wrinkles. It also removes toxins from the body to help reveal clearer skin.

INGREDIENTS

- 1 apple
- 2 cups strawberries
- A handful of kale leaves

PREPARATION

1. Remove the seeds from the apple and chop the strawberries into pieces. Take all these ingredients to the juicer and process them. Put the water at the end.
2. Mix well until you create a liquid consistency. Put this in a glass and enjoy.
3. Serving Size: Approximately 1 glass (8–10 oz)

Calories: 80-100 kcal
Total Fat: 0-1g
Saturated Fat: 0g

Cholesterol: 0mg
Sodium: 0-5mg
Total Carbohydrate: 20-25g

Dietary Fiber: 4-5g
Sugars: 14-18g
Protein: 1-2g

Ginger and Lemon Juice

Ginger is an ancient culinary ingredient whose benefits cannot be denied. It is a rich source of potassium and niacin, minerals necessary for your body. This wonderful vegetable helps you have healthy and radiant skin. This is great for skin problems as it contains 40 antioxidant compounds that protect the skin from premature aging, dullness, sagging skin, and acne scarring. It also helps eliminate toxins and increases blood circulation, which improves skin condition. Ginger juice is excellent, so adding lemon juice makes it even better.

INGREDIENTS

- 1 piece of ginger
- 2 tbsp lemon juice

PREPARATION

1. Slice the ginger and chop it into pieces. Extract lemon juice.
2. Take these ingredients to the juicer and put a little water in it.
3. Mix well so that you create a runny consistency.
4. Serving Size: Approximately 1 glass (8–10 oz)

Calories: 15-20 kcal
Total Fat: 0g
Saturated Fat: 0g

Cholesterol: 0mg
Sodium: 0-5mg
Total Carbohydrate: 4-5g

Dietary Fiber: 0-1g
Sugars: 1-2g
Protein: 0g

Pineapple, Cucumber, and Parsley Juice

Adding pineapple juice will make this healthy recipe even tastier. This ingredient is perfect for sensitive and inflamed skin, as it contains vitamin C, which helps heal and soothe. It is also a great source of antioxidants that soothe cell damage caused by free radicals and oxidative stress.

Parsley is a wonderful herb famous for healing the skin. It has a minty flavor and smell that is sure to refresh you after a hard day's work. It is rich in vitamins C and K, which are essential for producing collagen and maintaining skin elasticity. At the same time, it promotes smooth skin by increasing collagen production to aid in cell renewal and repair. It also controls sebum production, which calms acne and blackhead problems. Cucumber juice will serve to keep the body deeply hydrated and deeply nourishes the skin as it is rich in silica. Drink this juice daily for glowing skin.

INGREDIENTS

- 1 cucumber
- 1 pineapple
- A handful of parsley

PREPARATION

1. Slice the cucumber and cut it into pieces. Cut and peel the pineapple and leave it in cubes. Chop the parsley leaves as you like.
2. Place all the ingredients in the juicer. If it is too thick add ½ cup of water and mix for a few minutes until you have a smooth paste.
3. Serve in a glass and enjoy.
4. Serving Size: Approximately 1 glass (8–10 oz)

Calories: 100-120 kcal
Total Fat: 0.5-1g
Saturated Fat: 0g

Cholesterol: 0mg
Sodium: 10-20mg
Total Carbohydrate: 25-30g

Dietary Fiber: 3-4g
Sugars: 20-25g
Protein: 1-2g

Pure Aloe Vera Juice

Aloe vera juice is an all-rounder that can greatly improve the quality of your skin and hair. It is rich in vitamins and minerals to help maintain the skin's natural glow. It contains hormones like auxin and gibberellin, which are good for skin healing. It also has anti-inflammatory properties. You should drink this juice every morning for maximum glow.

INGREDIENTS

- A few stems of aloe vera

PREPARATION

1. Slice the aloe vera stems and chop them into chunks. Extract the sap from it.
2. Put it in a juicer. If it is thick, you can put ½ cup of water and combine for a few minutes until you have a liquid consistency.
3. Put it in a glass and enjoy. Consume these power-packed vegetable juices for seriously glowing skin and help with skin health naturally.

Calories: 0-5 kcal (may vary based on serving size)
Total Fat: 0g
Saturated Fat: 0g

Cholesterol: 0mg
Sodium: 0-10mg (depending on processing)
Total Carbohydrate:

0-1g (minimal)
Dietary Fiber: 0g
Sugars: 0-1g (minimal)
Protein: 0g

Broccoli, Kale, and Spinach Juice

INGREDIENTS

- A bouquet of broccoli flowers
- 1 kale
- A bunch of spinach

PREPARATION

1. Place all the ingredients in a juicer and blend until smooth.
2. Then pass them through a strainer.
3. Serve either cold or fresh and enjoy.
4. In the next chapter, I will show you a series of recipes that will boost your energy and make you feel refreshed and healthy. In addition, they are delicious and easy to make, like all the ones we have made so far.

Calories: 30-40 kcal (may vary based on serving size)
Total Fat: 0g
Saturated Fat: 0g

Cholesterol: 0mg
Sodium: 50-100mg (may vary based on ingredients and serving size)

Total Carbohydrate: 7-10g
Dietary Fiber: 3-4g
Sugars: 2-4g
Protein: 3-4g

CHAPTER 7
ENERGY BOOSTER JUICE RECIPES

Take note of these recipes to boost energy, these are delicious and will keep you strong and active all day.

In this chapter, I will show you how to increase energy, but remember, it is part of a boost to the process of recovering and boosting yourself. You will know some smoothie recipes that will help you combine and expand your options.

Green Apple Spinach Energizer

INGREDIENTS

- 1–2 ginger pieces
- 1 lemon, peeled
- 1 green apple
- 1 cucumber
- 2 cups spinach
- 2 kiwis
- 2 pineapple slices or a piece of watermelon

PREPARATION

1. Cut the ends (or butts) of each of the citrus fruits.
2. Stand the fruit upright on top of one flat end and slice down. Try not to cut the skin too much, or the juice will run out.
3. Chop down close to the entire citrus fruit until every rind is removed
4. For apples and cucumbers, keep the skin and chop them into four pieces.
5. Remove the skin from kiwis, pineapple, and/or watermelon. Chop the pineapple or watermelon into 1-inch cubes.
6. Pass each one through the juicer, combine, and enjoy.

Calories: 150-200 kcal (may vary based on serving size)
Total Fat: 1-2g
Saturated Fat: 0g

Cholesterol: 0mg
Sodium: 20-40mg (may vary based on ingredients and serving size)

Total Carbohydrate: 35-40g
Dietary Fiber: 6-8g
Sugars: 20-25g
Protein: 2-3g

Chocolate Banana Juice

A smoothie is another way to make a homemade energy shake for breakfast, but the preparation itself is more or less the same, just served on a plate. Therefore, we are going to start our list with this very special smoothie, setting the bar very high since it is a very energetic drink that is not too hard to make, with chocolate and banana all in one. Perfect for breakfasts and snacks!

INGREDIENTS

- ½ cup non-dairy milk
- 2 tbsp peanut butter
- 3 frozen bananas
- 5 tbsp cocoa powder
- **To decorate:**
- Chopped chocolate
- Dry fruit
- Banana slices
- Chia seeds
- This is one of the best energy shakes, and it is very easy to prepare if you follow the steps below.
- **Properties of This Smoothie**
- Cocoa powder. It has a lot of vegetable fat, but it is healthy and energizing. When you buy a chocolate bar, it should contain at least 70% cocoa so you can take advantage of its powerful antioxidants—even better if you buy it with little or no added sugar.
- Vegetable milk. These types of drinks are not only suitable for vegans and lactose intolerant people but also for people with slow digestion.
- Chia seeds. This food is rich in omega-3 fatty acids, proteins, and amino acids. Powerful energy!
- Chia seeds. Although they provide few carbohydrates, they contain a good amount of healthy fats and provide proteins of moderate biological value (it has a lot of arginines, but little lysine and methionine). Pure energy!
- Banana. It provides a variety of sugars, vitamins, and minerals.

PREPARATION

1. Place the juice ingredients in the blender after chopping them. When serving the mix, layer it with chocolate chunks, bananas, seeds, and other ingredients.
2. Orange and Mint Juice
3. Ingredients
4. 1 orange, peeled
5. 1/2 lemon, peeled
6. 1/4 inch fresh ginger root
7. 2-3 mint leaves
8. 4 carrots
9. Preparation
10. Wash each food well.
11. Take them to the juicer.
12. Process and serve it immediately.

Calories: Approximately 80-100 calories per serving.
Total Fat: Less than 1 gram per serving.
Saturated Fat: Negligible (virtually 0 grams).
Cholesterol: 0 milligrams per serving.
Sodium: Less than 10 milligrams per serving.
Total Carbohydrate: Approximately 20-25 grams per serving.
Dietary Fiber: Approximately 3-4 grams per serving.
Sugars: Approximately 10-15 grams per serving.
Protein: Approximately 1-2 grams per serving.

Oatmeal With Fruits Juice

Oats are excellent for fighting fatigue and prolonging our energy for longer because they contain slow and easy absorption of carbohydrates, which is why they are part of many energy shakes. Now, we've included it in this recipe, but with toppings like apples and bananas.

INGREDIENTS

- 1 tsp cinnamon
- 1 cup rolled oats
- 1 cup fresh strawberries
- 1 cup almond milk
- 2 bananas
- 2 green apples

PREPARATION

1. With the ingredients in hand, the next step is to cook the oats with 2 cups of water. When ready, let it cool and process in a blender along with the chopped strawberries.
2. Cube the apples and add the almond milk to the blender. Turn the machine back on and mix until all ingredients are combined.
3. Add chopped and mashed bananas at the end to complete your healthy smoothie. Add a splash of almond milk if you find it too thick.
4. Enjoy this smoothie by adding a pinch of ground cinnamon to each ready-to-drink glass.
5. This juice can be served cold with a little ice at room temperature. You can combine this energy drink with some energy bars with fruits.
6. **Properties of This Smoothie**
7. Apple. It's one of the most energy-providing fruits, but that doesn't mean it's calorie-dense and packed with plenty of micronutrients. It's good for electrolyte replacement after physical activity because it's high in potassium and its healthy sugar content stimulates endorphin production, which lifts your mood.
8. Strawberry. Its carbohydrates are in the form of fructose, glucose, and xylitol, but its caloric intake is very low. It provides a good amount of vitamin C, even more than an orange, and is full of antioxidants.
9. Banana. Its tryptophan content, a substance that is later converted into serotonin, has a positive effect on mood and relaxes the body.
10. Pomegranate, Orange, and Pineapple
11. Ingredients
12. ½ pomegranate
13. ½ cup pineapple
14. 1 orange
15. Preparation
16. Chop the pomegranate into 4 pieces and set aside the seeds in a bowl.
17. Peel the orange and remove the skin and core of the pineapple. Chop into appropriate sizes.
18. Place all the ingredients in the juicer.
19. When it comes out, serve it and enjoy.

Calories: Approximately 100-120 calories per serving.
Total Fat: Less than 1 gram per serving.
Saturated Fat: Negligible (virtually 0 grams).
Cholesterol: 0 milligrams

per serving.
Sodium: Less than 10 milligrams per serving.
Total Carbohydrate: Approximately 25-30 grams per serving.
Dietary Fiber: Approximately

4-6 grams per serving.
Sugars: Approximately 15-20 grams per serving.
Protein: Approximately 1-2 grams per serving.

Wild Smoothie

The secret of red fruits is that they provide a lot of energy and micronutrients, but they have a very low glycemic index and caloric intake; that's why they're often seen in juice recipes for energy. Here we are going to blend them with a banana and yogurt for a powerful and nutritious smoothie, but if you want to take it a little higher, you can add 2 crushed cookies or oatmeal. Highly recommended for those who train!

INGREDIENTS

- 2 bananas
- 2 boxes of blueberries
- 2 boxes of blackberries
- 500 ml strawberry yogurt

PREPARATION

1. Add bananas and strawberry yogurt to a blender glass.
2. Add the blackberries and mix.
3. Place the blueberries last.
4. Decorate with some blackberries and some blueberries on top.
5. **Other Properties of This Smoothie**
6. Yogurt. It contains 5% of our daily requirement of magnesium, an essential mineral for the nervous system to work and the reduction of fatigue. In addition, it provides us with group B vitamins, responsible for the proper functioning of the muscle system and the repair of injured muscles.
7. Orange Light
8. Ingredients
9. ¼ cup banana
10. ⅓ cup bok choy
11. ½ orange
12. 1 cup sliced oranges
13. Preparation
14. Peel the banana and orange and cut them into appropriate sizes.
15. Wash the bok choy leaves well and cut them into 2-inch pieces.
16. Place the ingredients in the juicer and process.
17. Enjoy! Pour over ice, if desired.

Calories: Approximately 80-100 calories per serving.
Total Fat: Less than 1 gram per serving.
Saturated Fat: Negligible (virtually 0 grams).
Cholesterol: 0 milligrams per serving.
Sodium: Less than 10 milligrams per serving.
Total Carbohydrate: Approximately 20-25 grams per serving.
Dietary Fiber: Approximately 3-5 grams per serving.
Sugars: Approximately 10-15 grams per serving.
Protein: Approximately 1-2 grams per serving.

Mango and Almond Smoothie

Mangoes are another great source of carbohydrates in the fruit, after bananas and grapes. For this reason, fruit smoothies containing mango are a favorite among athletes, but they are also great for children and anyone who has a heavy job or is sick. Ideal for breakfast or as a snack!

INGREDIENTS

- 1 tbsp lemon juice
- 1 tbsp ground almonds
- 1 tsp vanilla extract
- 1 large mango
- 1 handful of ice
- 125 ml skimmed natural yogurt
- 2 tbsp honey
- 250 ml skimmed milk

PREPARATION

1. To make this mango almond juice, start by peeling and dicing the mango.
2. In a blender, put chopped mango, ground almonds, skimmed milk, yogurt, vanilla essence, lemon juice, and honey. Mix until there is a homogeneous compound without lumps.
3. Finally, separate the mango milkshakes into two glasses with a little ice, pour, and serve.
4. You have now prepared a fabulous mango and almond smoothie perfect for sharing.
5. **Properties of This Smoothie**
6. Skimmed milk. Casein, the main milk protein, is slowly absorbed due to its sustained and prolonged release of amino acids between 7-8 hours, which is necessary for the recovery and maintenance of muscle mass, especially at night (avoid catabolism) to build muscle. Skim milk and yogurt are recommended for those who want to lose weight.
7. Non-fat plain yogurt. It is more digestible than milk because it contains less lactose, so it is better absorbed by the body. In addition, its high-quality serum protein and casein protein provide effects such as satiety, muscle growth, and protection of the bone system.
8. Honey. Its carbohydrate composition is mainly based on fast-absorbing simple sugars (glucose and fructose). Pure fast energy! What is the biggest difference between honey and refined sugar? Although their caloric intake is very similar, sugar is devoid of calories, while honey provides: mineral salts, vitamins, proteins, and enzymes.
9. Tip: Mangoes provide high amounts of fiber in doses comparable to bananas and kiwis, which facilitate intestinal transit and regulate glucose.
10. Lemon Berry
11. Ingredients
12. 1/3 lemon
13. 1/3 cup kiwi
14. 1/3 cup white grapes
15. 2 cups whole strawberry
16. Preparation
17. Peel and cut the kiwi and lemon into appropriate sizes.
18. Remove the white grapes from the stem and the stems from the strawberries and wash them properly.
19. Put the white grapes in the juicer along with the kiwi, strawberries, and lemon.
20. Add ice if you want.

Calories: Approximately 70-90 calories per serving.
Total Fat: Less than 1 gram per serving.
Saturated Fat: Negligible (virtually 0 grams).

Cholesterol: 0 milligrams per serving.
Sodium: Less than 10 milligrams per serving.
Total Carbohydrate: Approximately 17-20 grams per serving.

Dietary Fiber: Approximately 3-5 grams per serving.
Sugars: Approximately 10-13 grams per serving.
Protein: Approximately 1-2 grams per serving

Peanut Butter and Banana Juice

This drink is ideal for breakfast, as a snack, or after training. If you want to boost your energy, add oatmeal, crackers, or a sugar-free cereal. If you just want to pair it with breakfast, you can finish the meal with a veggie sandwich and some protein (chicken or tuna).

INGREDIENTS

- 2 banana or plantain
- 50 ml milk
- 2 tbsp peanut butter

PREPARATION

1. Prepare each of the ingredients to make this delicious peanut butter and banana juice.
2. Freeze a cut and peeled banana. Once it's completely frozen, you can take it to a blender and grind it up. Help yourself with a spatula to make the process easier.
3. Then add the milk a little at a time and continue adding the banana-peanut smoothie.
4. Place the peanut butter and mix. The result should be a thick and creamy shake.
5. Other Properties of This Smoothie
6. Peanut butter is very energizing because it is rich in fatty acids and protein. In addition, it promotes muscle recovery while exercising, thanks to its magnesium content, B vitamins, and antioxidants (polyphenols). As if that were not enough, it also provides us with fiber, tryptophan, and other bioactive compounds, making it a potentially healthy food.
7. Bananas are the favorite fruit of athletes and children, followed by apples. It is high in carbohydrates, potassium, and magnesium; they explain themselves since it is one of the most common fruits in juice recipes for energy.
8. Tip: Although peanuts are classified as a nut, they are a legume that grows in a pod.
9. Lemon, Carrot, and Orange Juice
10. Ingredients
11. 2 oranges
12. 4 carrots
13. Small ginger
14. 1/2 lemon
15. Preparation
16. Cut and peel the lemons and oranges into slices.
17. Peel and chop the carrot and ginger.
18. Place all the ingredients in the juicer.

Calories: Approximately 80-100 calories per serving.
Total Fat: Less than 1 gram per serving.
Saturated Fat: Negligible (virtually 0 grams).

Cholesterol: 0 milligrams per serving.
Sodium: Less than 10 milligrams per serving.
Total Carbohydrate: Approximately 20-25 grams per serving.

Dietary Fiber: Approximately 3-5 grams per serving.
Sugars: Approximately 15-20 grams per serving.
Protein: Approximately 2-3 grams per serving.

Strawberry and Kiwi Juice

Kiwis and strawberries fight fatigue, increase energy and improve mood, which is why they are among the favorite fruits of athletes. Now, if you want your drink to be one of your favorite recipes to lose weight with energy shakes, drink it 3 times a week before breakfast and, occasionally, as a substitute for your first meal of the day. Of course, to lose weight, this drink can be prepared with skimmed or vegetable milk and without adding sugar.

INGREDIENTS

- ½ cup strawberries
- 1 cup oats
- 1 cup ice
- 1 cup milk (240 ml)
- 3 kiwis
- 35 g (1.2 oz) sugar (optional)

PREPARATION

1. The first step you must take to prepare this strawberry and kiwi smoothie is to have all the ingredients ready.
2. Peel the kiwi and cut it into pieces.
3. Chop the strawberries, add the kiwi, add the sugar, and put the mix in the refrigerator for 10 minutes.
4. To continue making the strawberry and kiwi smoothie, add the previous mixture to a blender along with 1 cup of milk and blend.
5. Then, add ice and blend again so that your smoothie is super frozen.
6. Serve and enjoy this delicious strawberry and Kiwi ice cream shake.

Calories: Approx. 150-180 cal
Total Fat: Approx. 3-5 g
Saturated Fat: Approx. 1-2 g
Cholesterol: < 5 mg

Sodium: < 50 mg
Total Carbohydrate: Approx. 30-35 g
Dietary Fiber: Approx. 4-6 g

Sugars: Approx. 10-15 g
Protein: Approx. 5-7 g

Grapefruit, Carrot, and Ginger

INGREDIENTS

- A 1-inch fresh ginger
- 2 grapefruits
- 5 small carrots

PREPARATION

1. Chop and peel the grapefruits and ginger as they will fit in the juicer.
2. Place all the ingredients in the appliance and process.
3. Serve immediately.

Calories: Approx. 80-100 cal
Total Fat: < 1 g
Saturated Fat: < 1 g
Cholesterol: 0 mg

Sodium: 40-60 mg
Total Carbohydrate: Approx. 20-25 g
Dietary Fiber: Approx. 4-6 g

Sugars: Approx. 10-12 g
Protein: Approx. 2-3 g

Green Juice With Banana

This vibrant green smoothie gets its color from spinach and avocado, two remarkable foods that fight fatigue and restore energy. Avocado reduces bad cholesterol and favors the repair of muscle mass. Thanks to its healthy fats and micronutrients, among the latter, several B vitamins and potassium stand out, with more doses than bananas. As for spinach, it's not exactly a powerhouse vegetable, but its rich nutritional profile complements the dish nicely.

INGREDIENTS

- ½ avocado
- 1 tbsp oat flakes
- 1 tsp flower honey
- 1 banana
- 150 g spinach
- 250 ml milk

PREPARATION

1. Gather all the ingredients.
2. Peel and chop the banana and place it in a blender glass with the milk.
3. Add the rolled oats and beat with a mixer.
4. Place the washed and diced spinach and continue beating until there are no lumps.
5. Then, add the avocado you previously peeled. Avocado gives a creamy texture to this green smoothie.
6. Finally, add 1 teaspoon of nectar to sweeten this power shake while adding even more nutrition.
7. If the green banana smoothie is too thick, add a few ice cubes or add a little more milk.

Calories: Approx. 250-300 cal
Total Fat: 11-12 g
Saturated Fat: 2-3 g
Cholesterol: 0 mg

Sodium: 80-100 mg
Total Carbohydrate: Approx. 35-40 g
Dietary Fiber: Approx. 7-9 g

Sugars: Approx. 15-18 g
Protein: Approx. 6-8 g

Tofu Smoothie

If you're vegan, lactose intolerant, or just want to try other things and look for an energy shake to exercise with, then this is something you'll want. On this occasion, we use tofu to replace the protein part of animal origin since this food is rich in proteins of high biological value and provides 8 types of essential amino acids for the human organism, plus the potassium from the oranges and mangoes, the carbs from the mangoes, the healthy fats and protein from the almonds, and all the micronutrients present in all the ingredients. This is one of the best prepared-at-home shakes to boost energy and defense with just a few ingredients.

INGREDIENTS

- 1 orange
- 50 g (1.7 oz) almonds
- 80 g (2.8 oz) natural semi-hard tofu
- 100 g (3.5 oz) mango

PREPARATION

1. Before making this energy shake, the first step is to prepare all the ingredients.
2. In a blender, process the orange juice and the mango, peeled and cut into cubes, until obtaining a homogeneous mixture.
3. Add the almonds and tofu and mix again to combine.
4. Lastly, add ice cubes. This drink has no added sugar and you can add some if you wish.
5. Serve a tofu smoothie, perfect for cereal or post-workout granola bars.

Calories: Approx. 300-350 cal
Total Fat: 18-20 g
Saturated Fat: 2-3 g
Cholesterol: 0 mg

Sodium: 0-5 mg
Total Carbohydrate: Approx. 30-35 g
Dietary Fiber: Approx. 6-8 g

Sugars: Approx. 20-25 g
Protein: Approx. 10-12 g

Apple and Walnuts Juice

For those looking for a healthy dairy-free smoothie, you will love this recipe, not only for its nutritional content but also for its delicate flavor profile. Remember, when you're making a nutrient-dense breakfast shake, it's best to include long-lasting carbohydrates, in which case you can add 1 cup of oats as an extra ingredient. At dinner, it is used to build muscle mass while you sleep, in which case oatmeal is optional.

INGREDIENTS

- 1 apple
- 1 pinch of ground cinnamon
- 300 ml milk or non-dairy milk (1 ¼ cups)
- 304 g walnuts
- To decorate:
- 1 handful of pine nuts

PREPARATION

1. Prepare all the ingredients.
2. In a blender glass, place the nuts, apple, milk, and cinnamon.
3. Blend the apple-walnut smoothie until smooth. You can strain your smoothie to make it smoother and taste better.
4. This apple and walnut smoothie can be garnished with some pine nuts on top.
5. On the other hand, peel and cut the apples. Put these pieces in a blender glass and cover them with milk. Note that if you are lactose intolerant, you have the option of using almond milk or soy milk, but note that the flavor will vary depending on which product you choose.

Calories: Approx. 450-500 cal
Total Fat: 40-45 g
Saturated Fat: 3-4 g
Cholesterol: 0 mg

Sodium: 0-5 mg
Total Carbohydrate: Approx. 15-20 g
Dietary Fiber: Approx. 4-6 g

Sugars: Approx. 8-12 g
Protein: Approx. 10-12 g

Banana and Orange Smoothie

INGREDIENTS

- 1 tsp honey
- 1 banana
- 2 oranges

PREPARATION

1. To make this natural energy drink, the first step to take is to peel and cut the banana. Keep in mind that you can use very ripe bananas, as this banana smoothie recipe is perfect for taking advantage of fruit that is about to go bad.
2. Also, squeeze the oranges until all the juice is removed.
3. Put all the fruit in the glass of the blender or juicer you normally use to make juice. Mix everything and add some honey. The idea is that the liquid juice does not have lumps.
4. Serve the banana-orange smoothie, and if you're craving a breakfast of champions, pair it with some yogurt muffins for a vitamin-packed breakfast.

Calories: Approx. 200-250 cal
Total Fat: Less than 1 g
Saturated Fat: Less than 1 g
Cholesterol: 0 mg

Sodium: Less than 1 mg
Total Carbohydrate: Approx. 50-60 g
Dietary Fiber: Approx. 6-7 g

Sugars: Approx. 35-40 g
Protein: Approx. 2-3 g

Avocado Green Juice

Avocado is a very tasty fruit that can help reduce cholesterol and triglyceride levels, and it is one of the richest foods in vitamin E.

INGREDIENTS

- ½ tsp fresh ginger
- 1 avocado
- 1 banana
- 100 ml coconut water

PREPARATION

1. Place all the ingredients to make the avocado green smoothie. In addition to avocados, coconut water also contains many vitamins, minerals, and antioxidants.
2. First, place the peeled bananas in the blender jar along with the fresh ginger (which we peeled before). The amount of ginger depends on your taste, so we recommend adding a small amount, trying making smoothies, and increasing as needed.
3. Next, peel the avocado. Remove the stone from the center, and place it in the glass of the blender.
4. It's time to add the coconut water. If you don't like it or want to reduce the coconut flavor, you can replace it with water or mix it in equal parts.
5. Blend the avocado green smoothie with the help of a blender until it has a fine texture and no lumps. Add more water or coconut water if necessary.
6. This drink is perfect for the morning before work. You will see the energy that this green avocado smoothie gives you!

Calories: Approx. 250-300 cal
Total Fat: Approx. 13-15 g
Saturated Fat: Approx. 2-3 g
Cholesterol: 0 mg
Sodium: Approx. 25-30 mg
Total Carbohydrate:

Approx. 35-40 g
Dietary Fiber: Approx. 8-10 g
Sugars: Approx. 15-20 g
Protein: Approx. 3-4 g
Vitamin E: Abundant
(from avocado)

Vitamin C: Moderate (from avocado and banana)
Potassium: High (from avocado and banana)

Coconut and Papaya Juice

We all love to have a refreshing drink close at hand on a hot day, and it's even better when it's natural and homemade. Fruit shakes, as you already know, have many vitamins that satisfy the appetite and provide us with a good amount of vitamins that are very necessary for our health.

INGREDIENTS

- ½ lime
- ½ papaya
- 1 banana
- 2 carrots
- 200 ml coconut water
- 350 ml water

PREPARATION

1. Gather all the ingredients to make this juice. Papaya, a tropical fruit with antioxidant and cleansing properties, is ideal for juices.
2. Peel the carrots, cut them into thin slices, and place them in a blender. Similarly, cut the papaya in half, remove the seed from the center, peel it, and add it to the blender.
3. Blend the papaya juice and add the juice of ½ lime. Continue beating so that the flavors melt. If you don't have limes, you can replace them with lemons, although the former is always more citrusy and have a very refreshing aroma.
4. Add the peeled bananas and continue stirring until all lumps are removed. If you prefer sweeter juice, you can add another banana to make it more delicious.
5. Put coconut fiber water and cold water until you get your favorite texture. Yogurt can also be added, but the smoothie will be thicker.
6. This coconut and papaya smoothie can be enjoyed for breakfast, as a snack, or between meals.

Calories: Approx. 150-200 cal
Total Fat: Approx. 1-2 g
Saturated Fat: Approx. 0.5 g
Cholesterol: 0 mg
Sodium: Approx. 30-40 mg
Total Carbohydrate:

Approx. 35-40 g
Dietary Fiber: Approx. 6-8 g
Sugars: Approx. 20-25 g
Protein: Approx. 2-3 g
Vitamin A: High (from papaya and carrots)

Vitamin C: Very High (from papaya and lime)
Vitamin B6: Moderate (from banana)
Potassium: High (from papaya and banana)

Oatmeal and Mango Juice

If you want to start your day off with a delicious breakfast, it can be fun managing a variety of options when it comes to your first meal of the day. When preparing breakfast, you should always consider including carbohydrates, proteins, and fruits to provide the body with a good energy base.

INGREDIENTS

- 1 tbsp honey
- 1 mango
- 1 pinch of refined sugar, brown sugar, or sweetener (optional)
- 1 cup instant oats
- 1 cup ice (optional)
- 1 ½ cup skimmed milk

PREPARATION

1. Put all the ingredients you need on the table to make this nutritious and refreshing oatmeal and mango smoothie.
2. Pour the milk and the peeled mango into a blender. Blend until the ingredients come together.
3. Mix the remaining ingredients in a blender, that is, the oats, honey, sugar, and ice. Remember, sugar and ice are optional. You can even add a bit of cinnamon if you like.
4. If the mixture is too thick, add more ice or milk. On the contrary, if it is liquid, put more oats, honey, and sugar. It all depends on your taste. Mix until obtaining a homogeneous liquid.
5. Refreshing and delicious! This oatmeal and mango smoothie is perfect for a quick and nutritious breakfast.

Calories: Approx. 250-300 cal
Total Fat: Approx. 2-3 g
Saturated Fat: Approx. 0.5 g
Cholesterol: 2-4 mg (from milk)
Sodium: Approx. 40-50 mg

Total Carbohydrate: Approx. 55-60 g
Dietary Fiber: Approx. 6-8 g
Sugars: Approx. 30-35 g
Protein: Approx. 7-9 g

Vitamin A: High (from mango)
Vitamin C: Very High (from mango)
Folic Acid: Moderate (from milk)
Iron: Moderate (from oats)

Oatmeal and Banana Juice

There are no excuses... have breakfast! Everyone knows that breakfast is essential for the body to function well throughout the day. However, many people also believe that if they skip this meal, they will lose weight quickly. The reality is quite different, because if you don't eat your first meal of the day, your body suffers, and also your metabolism slows down, which can lead to weight gain.

INGREDIENTS

- ½ cup whole grain oats
- 1 banana, ripe is much better
- 1 pinch of natural honey (to taste)
- 1 cup plain low-fat or Greek yogurt
- 4 ice cubes (or to taste)
- 4 tsp flax seeds
- Non-fat soy milk or rice milk

PREPARATION

1. To get started with this oatmeal smoothie recipe for weight loss, start by laying out the ingredients on the table. Measure, weigh, and reserve all the ingredients before starting. Pour all the components into a blender and blend at high speed. This is a very simple, healthy, and delicious drink! If you want your oatmeal and banana smoothie to be a little more natural, make your own soy or rice milk.
2. Serve this smoothie, garnish with flaxseed, and enjoy! This is an ideal drink to achieve the desired figure or maintain a line.

Calories: Approx. 350-400 cal
Total Fat: Approx. 5-7 g
Saturated Fat: Approx. 1-2 g
Cholesterol: 0 mg (if using non-fat soy or rice milk)
Sodium: Approx. 50-60 mg
Total Carbohydrate: Approx. 65-70 g
Dietary Fiber: Approx. 9-11 g
Sugars: Approx. 20-25 g
Protein: Approx. 15-17 g

Oatmeal, Honey, and Amaranth Juice

INGREDIENTS

- 1 lb almond milk
- 150 g (5.3 oz) oat flakes
- 40 ml honey
- 60 g (2.11 oz) amaranth seeds
- 2 tbsp peanut butter

PREPARATION

1. The first step to making this nutritious natural juice recipe is to prepare the ingredients.
2. Heat a skillet over a medium flame and toast the amaranth seeds until they turn a dark brown color. Once toasted, reserve them to use later in recipes. Keep in mind that amaranth seeds contain various properties derived from plants, such as calcium that helps prevent osteoporosis.
3. Place the oats and almond milk in a bowl and process the two ingredients until fully combined.
4. To give extra flavor to your shake, add peanut butter. If you don't have peanut butter, you can add almond butter for a special touch.
5. Put amaranth seeds and honey at the end, which will sweeten the smoothie.
6. Serve with lots of ice for a refreshing boost.

Calories: Approx. 450-500 cal
Total Fat: Approx. 15-20 g
Saturated Fat: Approx. 2-3 g
Cholesterol: 0 mg

Sodium: Approx. 100-150 mg
Total Carbohydrate: Approx. 70-75 g
Dietary Fiber: Approx. 7-9 g

Sugars: Approx. 20-25 g
Protein: Approx. 10-12 g

Apple and Banana Smoothie

INGREDIENTS

- 1 cup milk (240 ml)
- 1 red apple
- 1 banana
- 1/2 oz sugar

PREPARATION

1. For this healthy apple and banana smoothie, you have to add all the ingredients.
2. Chop the apples and put them in a blender along with half the sugar.
3. Peel and cut the banana and add it to the blender along with the remaining half of the sugar.
4. Mix with the milk until the mixture is liquid.
5. Serve and enjoy a banana–apple smoothie with a dash of cinnamon.

Calories: Approx. 220-250 cal
Total Fat: Approx. 2-3 g
Saturated Fat: Approx. 1-1.5 g
Cholesterol: Approx.

5-10 mg (from milk)
Sodium: Approx. 30-40 mg
Total Carbohydrate: Approx. 50-55 g

Dietary Fiber: Approx. 6-7 g
Sugars: Approx. 35-40 g
Protein: Approx. 4-5 g

Blueberry Banana Smoothie

Blueberry Banana Smoothie is a delicious way to energize the body, burn calories, and provide our daily serving of fruit. Although there is nothing mysterious about it, the mixture of these fruits will give you a colorful and refreshing drink.

INGREDIENTS

- 1 glass of skimmed milk
- 1 small glass of blueberry
- 2 bananas

PREPARATION

1. Making a blueberry smoothie is very easy. First, prepare all your ingredients. Remember, you can substitute milk for yogurt, and you can use ripe bananas so you don't have to add sugar or sweeteners to your natural smoothies.
2. Peel and chop the bananas a bit, this will help mix everything up. It doesn't matter if the banana has brown parts or not.
3. Place all the ingredients in a blender and blend at maximum power until you get a slightly thick and homogeneous mixture.
4. When everything is crushed, have two glasses with a lot of ice ready. If you have a powerful blender, you can add ice directly to make a smoothie.
5. Pour the blueberry–banana smoothie and serve chilled. You don't need to add sugar, but you can add a bit of honey if you think it needs it.

Calories: Approx. 200-250 cal
Total Fat: Approx. 1-2 g
Saturated Fat: Approx. 0.5-1 g
Cholesterol: Approx.

5-10 mg (from milk)
Sodium: Approx. 30-40 mg
Total Carbohydrate:
Approx. 50-55 g

Dietary Fiber: Approx. 6-7 g
Sugars: Approx. 30-35 g
Protein: Approx. 4-5 g

Protein Shake With Banana and Nuts

Many of us are familiar with protein shakes ready to mix with water or other drinks, and while they are good, there is nothing better than consuming natural products, like this recipe, a home-made protein shake made from ingredients natural such as fruits and nuts.

INGREDIENTS

- 1 tsp sugar
- 1 banana
- 100 ml natural yogurt
- 2 unsalted crackers
- ½ oz walnuts
- 200 ml milk

PREPARATION

1. Before making this homemade protein shake, the first step is to prepare all the ingredients. For this shake, we're going to use unsalted crackers.
2. Place milk, yogurt, and peeled and diced banana in a blender. Process until a homogeneous mixture is obtained.
3. Add the nuts, cookies, and sugar. Process again until a homogeneous mixture is obtained.
4. Finish with the protein shake served with bananas and walnuts. You can take this drink after your daily exercise routine.

Calories: Approx. 350-400 cal
Total Fat: Approx. 15-20 g
Saturated Fat: Approx. 3-4 g
Cholesterol: Approx. 10-
15 mg (from yogurt)
Sodium: Approx. 150-200 mg
Total Carbohydrate:
Approx. 40-45 g
Dietary Fiber: Approx. 3-4 g
Sugars: Approx. 25-30 g
Protein: Approx. 12-15 g

Mango Lassi Juice

Lassi is a traditional Indian drink made from yogurt and milk. Known for its cooling power, Lassi can be made salty, sweet, or spicy, all of which are perfect with any type of food, especially those with a strong flavor. With this recipe, we are going to teach you how to make a mango smoothie, one of the most popular smoothies in the West, which you can also have as a dessert.

INGREDIENTS

- 1 pinch of cardamom powder
- 130 ml milk
- 2 tsp sugar
- 7 oz mango
- 250 ml natural yogurt

PREPARATION

1. Making mango lassi is very simple, the important thing is that the raw material is good. For the mangoes, I advise you to use sweet mangoes, you will need about 3 if you are up for it. You can also use mango pulp.
2. Crush the mango completely, making sure that there are no lumps. Then mix with yogurt and milk.
3. Once you have your base mix ready, all you have to do is add sugar and a pinch of cardamom. The latter will give your shake a light taste and various health benefits.
4. Store in the fridge so the mango lassi is fresh and ready to enjoy. In India, this drink is served with meals, like traditional samosas or vegetable pakora, but it can also be eaten as a dessert.

Calories: Approx. 250-300 cal
Total Fat: Approx. 2-4 g
Saturated Fat: Approx. 1-2 g
Cholesterol: Approx. 10-
15 mg (from yogurt)
Sodium: Approx. 80-100 mg
Total Carbohydrate:
Approx. 45-50 g
Dietary Fiber: Approx. 2-3 g
Sugars: Approx. 40-45 g
Protein: Approx. 8-10 g

CONCLUSION

Fruit smoothies can help improve your health, are easy to prepare, and provide all the nutrients your body needs. Eating whole foods like fruits and vegetables will help improve brain function and promote healthy weight loss. As if that weren't enough, it also builds a stronger immune system in your body, allowing it to fight many diseases.

While you don't always have time to boil vegetables or prepare fruit dishes, the truth is that fruit juices are quick to make and can be enjoyed anytime, anywhere. Previously, I already told you some of the reasons why you should drink fruit juices and you now know all the benefits they provide.

If you drink juiced fruit smoothies regularly, you can boost your immune system and give your body more defense against foreign substances that can make you sick. In addition, the fruit will also help make your brain stronger and more receptive to information.

The good thing about fruit is that it fills you up between meals and you will be eating healthy. This is ideal especially when you have to lose weight or want to cleanse your body. Fruit juices can be a great way to help you lose weight, as long as you choose fruits that don't make you gain weight.

Some people replace meals with squeezed fruit juices, but you can do it once a day to cleanse your body. Juicing is not for you to do every day. To stay healthy, your body needs a varied and balanced diet to get all the essential nutrients and vitamins. We repeat: Once a day is fine, but no more. Fruit juices are ideal as a snack or in the morning.

The best part is that you have a plenty variety of fruits available so you can easily find a fruit combination that works for you. You will be able to discover many new flavors and enjoy delicious juices. Do you already know what fruits to mix to squeeze?

Give your morning a 180-degree turn: take out your juicer and start juicing the fruits you like. Add a little almond, coconut, or rice milk for a different and more nutritious flavor. You can also use different spices, herbs, and even different sweeteners to get the "best mix." Some shakes, such as *bananarama*, taste extraordinary due to the balanced mix of ingredients.

E. coli, Taenia solium, and Entamoeba histolytica have one thing in common: they are all microbes that, due to cross-contamination, can be found on fruits, vegetables, spices, and even in your extractor. Before making any juice or smoothie, remember to wash and disinfect the fruits and vegetables and the removable parts of your juicer. In this way, you can enjoy your drinks without having stomach problems. Also, consume juices and smoothies within the first 20 minutes of making them, as they then begin to lose mass and oxidize due to enzymes like polyphenol oxidase, thus depleting nutrients and reducing the appearance.

If you can't consume it right away, pour it into a container with minimal air and refrigerate for up to 3 days. When you need a drink to lift you, grab it straight from the fridge to keep you energized and refreshed.

Make the most of the fiber. Fruits and vegetables are rich in sugars, minerals, vitamins, and fiber. The latter exists in soluble and insoluble forms. Soluble fiber is found in oats, barley, nuts, seeds, and certain legumes; eating it helps slow the absorption of glucose and LDL or bad cholesterol.

Insoluble fiber, for its part, helps the body to evacuate and improves the digestive system, you can find it in peels and seeds, as well as in some tissues of fruits and vegetables. If you want all the benefits of fiber in one drink, blend the ingredients instead of juicing. Smoothies like soft tuna are high in soluble and insoluble fiber.

Eliminate oxalates. When making juices and smoothies, vary the topping mix because vegetables like spinach, kale, or beets are high in oxalates, minerals that can limit calcium absorption. Blanching these vegetables in antioxidant-power juices can reduce oxalate levels by up to 87%.

A glass of juice is not enough. Juices allow you to eat a variety of foods from different food groups in one glass. However, these can never replace a diet of a variety of solid foods, including oilseeds, vegetables, fruits, grains, dairy products, fats, and animal foods. If you like to supplement and change your routine, from time to time you can try a full low-calorie breakfast to keep you satisfied until lunchtime.

Prepare what you like, enjoy it, and get the most out of each ingredient.

BONUS 2: TIPS ON HOW TO SAVE MONEY BUYING ORGANIC FRUITS AND VEGETABLES

Introduction

Below you will see how to save money buying fruits and vegetables with general tips you can apply every time you prepare any of the recipes to take care of your body, although you can consider them to purchase other organic products.

We have been seeing in the previous chapters a series of juice recipes to use daily, either to lose weight, rejuvenate, feel radiant skin, or a series of other attributes.

Anyone who has been to an organic food store recognizes that organic foods tend to be a bit more expensive than conventional foods. However, there is a good reason behind most prices, and many times the extra cost is worth it.

Beware of Fake Organic Foods

The popularity of organic food has given rise to scammers; a person or company who sells non-organic and unsustainable products under false green credentials. This situation has considerably increased the number of cases of food fraud.

There is a big difference between genuine organic products and counterfeit organic products. True organic products are certified to meet higher quality control standards, which justifies the higher cost. Counterfeit organic products bypass these filters, using only the term organic as a hook to attract consumers and increase their value.

Since organic foods have audit trails and traceability certificates, fraud incidents are relatively rare compared to conventional foods. The most beneficial way to avoid falling into the trap and buying counterfeit organic products is to read the labels carefully, looking for the organic seal and the country of origin.

Don't Buy More Than You Need

Avoid improvisation preparing your weekly menu. Planning your regular menu, in addition to saving and buying responsibly, can help you follow healthier eating habits. Check your fridge and pantry before you shop, and consider the ingredients you'll need to set up your menu.

Beware of bargains or sales: Don't be tempted by sales, only take home necessary items. Remember, wasting food is wasting money.

Don't shop hungry. Shopping hungry has been shown to increase the number of items in your cart, most of which you don't need. No matter what you buy, including organic, these tips will keep you from wasting food and labor.

Organization

It's easy to overspend when you're cluttered. For example, buying pasta without checking the pantry because we already have the package. These oversights lead to much food being wasted. For this, the organization and labeling of leftovers are essential. If you're not methodical, it's time to get organized with these simple tips:

- Clean the pantry and the refrigerator at least every fortnight.
- Always label leftovers.
- Make food lists in the kitchen so you can check stocks.
- Use glass containers for leftovers.
- Organize your pantry logically. Baked products together, canned products together, etc.

Look for the Organic Seal

As consumers, we must know what we eat and take responsibility for choosing the best options for our lifestyles.

Always look for organic or eco stamps to avoid counterfeit organic food. However, some "organic" farms are indeed too small to afford certification. This would be an exception, in those cases, you would have to talk to the grower and see firsthand how they grow their products.

See the Long-Term Benefits

Eating organic products will not make you prettier or taller. You must understand that paying a little more for this type of product is a long-term investment. One way to save money on organic food is to trim your budget by cutting other household expenses. There are many ways to save money, such as reducing phone bills and avoiding subscriptions to pay TV channels you won't use in the future. Avoid buying very expensive bottled water whenever possible.

Cooking at home is usually the best solution to taking prepared meals to work; these are healthier and cheaper than in restaurants.

Join a Food Cooperative in Your Area

By joining a local food cooperative, you can get special discounts and save a lot of money. Generally, food cooperatives are created to support local farmers and other businesses in the area. While you don't have to be a member to buy products in a cooperative, the discounts are often higher if you are.

You can find advertising for food cooperatives in local magazines or at your local town hall.

Look at Seasonal Foods

Seasonal products are much cheaper. To find out which fruits are in season, look for a good seasonal food guide or ask at your trusted organic food store.

Seasonal foods—whether organic or not—are grown when weather conditions are right and plants are not forced to produce and are harvested at maturity according to their natural calendar. For great chefs and expert gourmets, seasonal fruits and vegetables are ideal for quality dishes due to their best organoleptic qualities: smell, taste, and texture.

Buy in Large Quantities

Getting food in bulk allows us to buy the size we want according to our needs. We can make a large monthly or yearly purchase and only keep large bags or boxes in the pantry for non-perishable items. But it also allows us to buy small quantities for smaller households, which is great for avoiding wasting food and creating more waste.

Apps for Savings

If receiving a coupon while paying makes you uncomfortable, don't worry, some apps can be your best friend because, with the help of your smartphone, you can take a photo of the receipt and choose which coupon is applied to that purchase discount. It's simple, fast, and super convenient.

See Offers

Every week, supermarkets offer product deals to attract more customers. To make the most of these deals, it's important to stay up-to-date by signing up for their deals newsletter and checking their brochures.

Take a tour of the sales area:

I am in the habit of shopping in the sale section first, as normally this area is used for products that no longer have their place on store shelves and are not replaced once they are gone. But since they are still in stock, the store is forced to move them away bundled with other products that met the same fate, and of course, lowered the price to get rid of them.

That is, you determine the maximum price you are willing to pay for an item you normally use so that you recognize a good opportunity. For example, it has happened to me that I do not cancel more than 1 dollar per pound of bananas, so when I see less than that, I take advantage and buy it without a problem.

Whatever You Buy, It Must Be of Quality

Many times we pay more for the same product because they sell us a brand image, but we can barely tell what it tastes like in blind tasting. There is almost no marketing or promotion of substandard fruits and vegetables. However, on blind taste, almost every customer would be able to tell the good tomatoes, apples, or bananas from the ordinary ones. High-quality fruits and vegetables are indeed healthier, even if they cost you a little more, it does not matter.

Trust an expert greengrocer in your area, and if it hasn't been tried yet, buy a little and then bigger baskets.

Start an Organic Home Garden

One way to save on organic food is to grow it on your patio or balcony. Get great, easy, and effective tips online on how to fertilize, control pests, and kill weeds without chemicals.

Final Tips for You to Save Money With Organic Food

- Do not buy pre-cooked foods; they are much more expensive than raw materials. It is best to cook in bulk organic products and freeze them later.
- Eat more parts of fruits and vegetables, including cauliflower and green stems, potato skins, and citrus peels. In this way, it is possible to take advantage of the benefits of organic products.
- Make a shopping list. If it's off the list, you're spending more than you want to.
- Buy cheaper organic cuts of meat to prepare stews or other more creative dishes. Also, consider eating less meat and preparing dishes with other protein-rich ingredients like lentils.
- Grow fruits and vegetables in your garden, even if it's just herbs on your windowsill or a cup of juicy tomatoes. Many books and sites can educate you on the instructions and materials you need to have your organic garden at home.
- Create an organic grocery shopping group to buy in bulk. You can find food at your local cooperative by searching online.

Conclusion

As for fruits, in some cases, you can buy what's fresh from the garden, so you can still enjoy those foods with the aroma they have when you separate them from the plant. Although it is good that you buy good food at affordable prices, I advise you to buy it in season and up to date.

BONUS 3: CREATIVE AND SIMPLE RECIPES TO USE THE LEFTOVER JUICE PULP

Introduction

These are some creative recipes you can make with the juice's leftover pulp, so you get the most out of every part of the fruit. You will be surprised by what you can do with something you usually throw away. I want to talk to you about how to use the leftover juice pulp, so we can waste less food and make something equally delicious with these ideas of using high-fiber pulp.

One of the most frequently asked questions about juice is "What can I do with the pulp of the juice?" A lot of things! Today we will take a look at 20 of my favorite uses for leftover juice pulp to inspire us to reduce food waste and make the most of the healthy fiber. Composting is an obvious choice, but there are other options for using juice pulp. Fortunately, we have discovered many unique recipes and methods over the years. Let's try them!

Broth for Soup

If you have never prepared your broth, this is your opportunity! I always like to make my broth and the pulp in the juice is the protagonist in this matter!

You can use fresh or frozen pulp in this recipe, just be sure to thaw it before doing so. I love making my vegetable broth—the pulp adds great flavor and some extra health benefits.

This broth can be used as a base for your favorite soup or stews you want to make, or you can enjoy it on its own! All you need is vegetable pulp, water, salt, pepper, and your favorite spices.

INGREDIENTS

- Vegetable pulp, the one you have left
- Salt to taste
- Water to taste
- Pepper to taste

PREPARATION

1. Pour 9-10 cups of water into a large pot and bring it to a boil.
2. When boiling, place all the vegetable pulp.
3. Season with salt, pepper, and whatever you have.
4. After adding the other ingredients, lower the heat to a simmer and cook for 45 minutes to 1 hour.
5. Let it cool a little.
6. Strain the remaining pulp or leave it in the broth, your choice!
7. Store in the refrigerator for up to 6 days and in the freezer for up to 3 months.

Vegan Basil Pesto Recipe

Here, we use the leftover pulp from cold-pressed almond milk to make a vegan basil pesto.

This pesto will keep for about 1 week in the fridge.

INGREDIENTS

- 8 tbsp extra-virgin olive oil
- 12 garlic cloves, peeled
- 2.5 oz basil
- 2.5 oz spinach
- Ground black pepper to taste
- Nut milk pulp, leftover from cold-pressed nut milk
- 1 tbsp salt
- Juice of 1/3 medium lemon

PREPARATION

1. In a frying pan, add the peeled garlic and cover with oil. I recommend that you use a small and shallow frying pan so you don't need too much oil to completely cover the garlic. Reduce heat to a simmer and simmer for 15-20 minutes, until the garlic is lightly golden and soft.
2. Remove the garlic from the oil and let both the garlic and the oil cool.
3. Add all ingredients except the oil to a blender and blend until well combined.
4. Little by little, add oil.

Apple Rice Pudding

INGREDIENTS

- 2 cups soy milk
- 1 cup apple pulp
- 1 cup apple juice
- 3 tbsp honey
- 1 tbsp finely chopped ginger root
- 1/2 cup yogurt
- 1/2 tsp ground cinnamon
- 1/2 tsp grated nutmeg
- 3/4 cup rice

PREPARATION

1. In a saucepan, combine the soy milk and rice. Bring it to a boil over medium-high heat. Cover, reduce heat, and simmer for 20 minutes or until rice is cooked but not tender.
2. Heating slightly, add the apple pulp, apple juice, and honey, and stir. Simmer for another 10 minutes or until the liquid has reduced slightly, the rice has softened, and the mixture has thickened. Remove from heat, add yogurt, ginger, cinnamon, and nutmeg, and stir.

Raw Pulp Cookies

We know that juice pulp cookies may not seem delicious at first, but these vegan and gluten-free cookies are sure to be a hit at your next event or gathering. They're tough enough to be added to any dip like hummus, guacamole, or spinach.

They are the perfect snack for those people with allergies or intolerances or those looking for something clean and healthy. You can use any vegetable pulp you like, but I prefer carrot pulp.

INGREDIENTS

- ¼ cup ground flax seeds
- ¼ cup quinoa flour
- ½ tsp sea salt
- ½ cup water
- 1 tbsp chia seeds
- 2 cups carrot juice pulp
- Sesame seeds

PREPARATION

1. The first thing that is needed is the pulp for the juice. It doesn't have to be just carrot juice. I guess beetroot juice will work too. But I have only tried recipes with carrots. You will need about 2 cups of pulp.
2. Place 2 cups of the pulp in a bowl along with 1/4 cup of ground flax seeds, 1 tablespoon of chia seeds, 1/4 cup of quinoa flour, and 1/2 teaspoon of salt. To keep it fresh, keep whole flaxseeds on hand and grind them in a coffee grinder. No flour is necessary, as the flax and chia seeds will hold the ingredients together.
3. Mix the ingredients so that the quinoa flour covers the carrot pulp well. Then let it rest for about 5 minutes. This is to allow the quinoa flowers to absorb the liquid from the carrot pulp.
4. This is where you have to work a little more. Depending on your juicer and how fresh the carrots are, you may need to improvise when adding water. Add half of the water, which is 1/4 cup, and mix. If you manage to form a ball and it sticks, it's done. The dough shouldn't be too sticky, but it shouldn't fall apart either. If you need more water, add 1 teaspoon at a time until desired results are achieved.
5. Let the dough rest for a while, then shape it into a disk. Put it on the parchment, place another piece on top, and roll out the dough to a thickness of 3 mm. You can adjust the thickness according to the type of cookies you want. If you make them thin, you can make chips to use in salads.
6. Sprinkle the top with chia and sesame seeds, pressing the seeds into the dough with parchment paper. Take a pizza cutter and cut the dough into cookie-sized pieces.
7. Place the dough still on the paper on a baking sheet and bake at 345°F for about 40 minutes. You will also need to adjust the moisture of the carrots. The cookies are ready when they no longer release when pressed. As the cookies bake, they shrink and separate.
8. Enjoy!

Applesauce

INGREDIENTS

- 1/2 tsp ground cinnamon
- 1/2 tsp grated nutmeg
- 2 cups filtered water
- 2 cups apple pulp
- 2 cups apple juice
- 3 tbsp honey

PREPARATION

1. In a nonreactive saucepan, combine the pulp, water, and juice. Bring it to a boil over medium-high heat.
2. Reduce heat to low and simmer for 20 to 30 minutes, or until the sauce thickens. Add honey, cinnamon, and nutmeg and stir. Serve warm or at room temperature. Store in an airtight container in the refrigerator.
3. Suggestion: Add 1/2 teaspoon (2 ml) of licorice powder for constipation, or 1/2 teaspoon (2 ml) of cayenne pepper or other herbs recommended for specific conditions.
4. To thicken or thin this compote, try adding carrot and beetroot juice with more or less water.

Cabbage Salad

INGREDIENTS

- 1 tbsp chopped dried apricot
- 1 cup carrot-apple pulp
- 1/2 cup chopped feta cheese, optional
- 1/2 cup of olive oil
- 2 tbsp soy sauce
- 2 tbsp flax seeds
- 2 tbsp raisins
- 2 tbsp freshly squeezed lemon juice
- 2 minced garlic cloves
- 2 cups cabbage pulp
- 3 tbsp sunflower seeds

PREPARATION

1. In a good-sized salad bowl, combine and toss the cabbage pulp, apple, carrot pulp, flaxseeds, sunflower seeds, and apricots.
2. In a small jar or bowl with a tight-fitting lid, combine the oil, lemon juice, soy sauce, and garlic. Shake or stir to mix well. Spread the dressing over the salad and toss to coat. Top with grated feta if desired.

Seasoning for Papaya Marinade

INGREDIENTS

- 1 cup papaya pulp
- 1 garlic clove, minced
- 1/2 cup soy sauce
- 2/3 cup freshly squeezed orange juice

PREPARATION

1. In a shallow baking dish, combine the pulp, orange juice, soy sauce, and garlic. Place the food to be marinated on a tray and cover both sides with a tablespoon of the marinade. Place it in the refrigerator for 1 hour, covered, turning once or twice. This marinade is delicious with fish and poultry.
2. Tip: If you don't have papaya pulp, use kiwi, orange, or pineapple pulp.

Avocado Gazpacho

INGREDIENTS

- 1 ripe avocado, chopped
- 1 tbsp chopped sweet
- 1 tbsp white wine vinegar
- Juice of 1 lemon
- 1/2 cucumber, seeded and chopped
- 2 garlic cloves
- 2 celery stalks, cut into chunks
- 2 cups vegetable pulp
- 2 cups vegetable or chicken broth
- 4 fresh basil or parsley sprigs

PREPARATION

1. In a food processor or blender, combine the broth, lemon juice, vinegar, pulp, celery, cucumber, garlic, basil, and avocado. Process it on high power until well blended (in two batches if necessary). Serve cool and garnish with hazelnut and fresh basil.
2. This rich summer gazpacho can be made with any vegetable puree.

Homemade Vinegar With Fruit Remains

You can use fruit remains, spoiled pieces, or bananas that have turned yellow. With them, you can make your own vinegar. That is the proposal of an expert chef in fermentation and waste reduction.

INGREDIENTS

- A non-metallic container
- Fruit
- Sugar
- Alongside the elements grows the aerobic acetic acid bacterium, Acetobacter. You require at least 7 oz of leftover fruit (skin, core, bruised whole fruit) and sugar or honey.

PREPARATION

1. Chop the fruit remains into small pieces and place them in a container.
2. On the scale, set the reading to zero, then cover the residue with cold water. Write down the weight of the water and add 1 tablespoon of sugar for every 9 oz of water.
3. Stir and cover with a cloth to allow the free flow of oxygen. Store at room temperature for a week out of direct sunlight, but stir daily.
4. Strain the fruit and let the liquid continue to ferment (always covered with a cloth) for 2–4 weeks. Finally, store it in a sterilized jar and it's ready to eat.

Cauliflower Stems With Tangerine Peel Sauce

This recipe encourages your imagination and creativity so as not to leave anything in the trash. That's what we do in this aromatic recipe, which uses cauliflower stems and orange zest with few additions.

INGREDIENTS

- 1 tsp honey
- 1 tsp mustard
- 1 tsp vinegar
- 1 pinch of olive oil
- 7 oz boiled potato
- 7 oz cauliflower stems
- Tangerine peel
- Salt to taste

PREPARATION

1. To prepare this recipe, the cauliflower stalks should be sliced very thin with a mandolin, and oil, vinegar, mustard, honey, and salt must be combined with the tangerine peel to make a vinaigrette.
2. The stems should be eaten raw, like a salad. Sprinkle 1 tablespoon of the sauce on a plate and make a salad with some boiled potato, freshly chopped stems, and a vinaigrette, says the chef. Season with fresh herbs if desired.

Pear and Apple Jelly

If you have accumulated 4 cups of apple and pear scraps, you can also use:

INGREDIENTS

- ¼ cup frozen or fresh cranberries
- ½ tsp fine sea salt
- 1 cup apple cider vinegar
- 1 cup sugar
- 2 cups apple cider vinegar

PREPARATION

1. In a saucepan with 2 cups of water, cook the peel and the remains of the apples, pears, or both with the other ingredients for half an hour, until the fruit falls apart easily. Pass it through a fine strainer over a bowl to collect the liquid; do not squeeze the rest, let it rest for a while so that it completely releases the water.

2. Pour the liquid back into the saucepan and cook over very low heat for about 20 minutes, until it has reduced by about three-quarters and large bubbles form. Let it cool and that's it. If it's too runny, you can reheat and reduce it a bit, but avoid caramelization.

You can store it in the fridge for up to 2 weeks or keep it in sterilized jars.

Baked Goods

Adding pulp from your juice to baked goods will add moisture to your favorite recipes. In some cases, you can even reduce the amount of olive oil or butter, use healthier alternatives, and make the most of the pulp.

Smoothies

Adding leftover pulp to a smoothie will give you additional nutrients and fiber. The pulp also helps thicken smoothies to a delicious consistency.

Experimenting is part of juicing, right? Have fun and try different combinations until you find your favorite, and you may even find your new beloved recipe!

Breakfasts

For a perfect breakfast stir-fry, fritters, or potatoes, add a few tablespoons of pulp from the juicer for added flavor. You can quickly prepare a nutritious breakfast in minutes.

Dehydrated Pulp

Nuts are a delicious dessert. You can easily make your own dried fruit using the pulp of fresh fruit. This is how you do it:

- Cover the cookie sheet with wax paper.
- Press and place the pulp evenly; make sure everything is level so everything dries at once.

- Put it in a dehydrator or the lowest part of the oven (preferably around 239°F) for 12-14 hours.
- Chop into strips and enjoy.

You can also mix lemon juice and/or sugar (depending on the sweetness of the fruit you want) with the pulp for a finer texture and sweeter flavor.

Ice Cream

Use the pulp you have left to make a delicious treat.

- Prepare the juice you like and save some for your ice cream.
- Sprinkle some of the pulp you have left in your ice cream molds.
- Pour the juice into the molds.
- Freeze and enjoy!

You can try a vast number of different flavors.

Cream Cheese Spread

Using the pulp from the juice, it's so easy to make your own cream cheese dip! It can be employed for cookies, sandwiches, and more.

Measure out about ½ cup of fruit or vegetable pulp (if using pulp, make sure the fruit is chopped or crushed).

Next, mix the pulp with about 1 cup of cream cheese. You can lightly beat the cream cheese by hand or with a mixer.

Salt and pepper the sauce to your liking. We recommend onion and garlic powder for mixed vegetables. Pop it in the fridge for about 2-4 hours to allow the flavors to meld and enjoy!

Edible Natural Dyes

You can use the leftover pulp to naturally make food coloring in different colors like yellow, green, red, purple, orange, and blue. This way you can enjoy your favorite dessert without compromising your health.

Dog Treats

Give love to your furry friend by making your healthy dog food with juice pulp.

INGREDIENTS

- ¼ cup ground flax
- ⅓ cup natural peanut butter
- ¾–1 ½ cup rolled oats
- 2 cups juice pulp
- Certain fruits and vegetables are bad for dogs. Please be careful they are not included in any of your treats.
- We recommend carrots, kale, cucumbers, apples (seedless), lettuce, celery, spinach, cantaloupe, and pears. Before preparing a treat, always make sure the ingredients are safe and healthy for your furry friend. If in doubt, consult your vet.

PREPARATION

1. Preheat the oven to 347°F.
2. Mix all the ingredients. Gradually pour in the rolled oats until you get a good dough consistency.
3. Then, use the mixture to form candy shapes.
4. Bake on a baking sheet for 50 to 60 minutes.

Other Uses of Fruit Pulp

- Blend the pulp into a smoothie to add fiber.
- Clothes dying. Did you know that fruit juice can be used to dye clothes?
- Boil the pulp with water, add spices such as cinnamon or ginger, cool, and filter to make "fruit tea."
- Use the pulp of the vegetables to increase the nutrient density of macaroni and cheese or pasta sauces, or layer them in lasagna.
- Use it for burgers or homemade veggie fritters. The pulp adds moisture, flavor, and nutrition.
- Use the pulp of a fruit or vegetable to add flavor, texture, and moisture to pancakes.
- Use the pulp for raw pizza dough.
- You can make jam.
- Dehydrate and use as breadcrumbs.
- Use it in homemade skin care recipes like scrubs, masks, and soaps.

Conclusion

The fruit pulp can be used the give more consistency to smoothies or to make cookies, soups, and other recipes you saw in this bonus. Start them up and get the most out of your recipes!

INDEX OF RECIPES

Made in the USA
Middletown, DE
13 June 2024